Caring for s
malnourish

Ann Ashworth and Ann Burgess

With help from Louise Sserunjogi and Elizabeth Poskitt

Based on training modules developed by Ann Ashworth, Thandi Puoane, David Sanders and Claire Schofield

MACMILLAN

AED
Academy for Educational Development

TALC

FOOD AND NUTRITION TECHNICAL ASSISTANCE

USAID

LONDON SCHOOL OF HYGIENE & TROPICAL MEDICINE

Macmillan Education
Between Towns Road, Oxford OX4 3PP
A division of Macmillan Publishers Limited
Companies and representatives throughout the world

www.macmillan-africa.com

ISBN 0 333 959 45 0

First published 2003

Designed by Sue Clarke
Illustrated by David Gifford
Cover design by Jim Weaver

This book is also on the CD-Rom *Caring for severely malnourished children.*

This publication was made possible through the support provided to the Food and Nutrition Technical Assistance (FANTA) Project by the Office of Health and Nutrition of the Bureau for Global Programs Field Support and Research at the US Agency for International Development, under terms of Cooperative Agreement No. HRN-A-00-98-00046-00 awarded to the Academy for Educational Development (AED). The opinions expressed herein are those of the authors and do not necessarily reflect the views of the US Agency for International Development.

Printed and bound in Malaysia

2007 2006 2005 2004 2003
10 9 8 7 6 5 4 3 2 1

Contents

Dedication

We dedicate this book to all nurses and other health workers who care for severely malnourished children especially those working with few resources and limited support.

Acknowledgements

This book is based on training modules developed for nurses in South Africa and we thank their authors, Thandi Puoane, David Sanders and Claire Schofield, for their input. We also used the management guidelines in *Management of severe malnutrition: a manual for physicians and other senior health workers* (World Health Organization, Geneva, 1999). The US Agency for International Development provided funding for the book through the Food and Nutrition Technical Assistance Project of the Academy for Educational Development. We thank Bruce Cogill and Annette Sheckler for facilitating this.

Our reviewers, Louise Sserunjogi in Uganda and Dr Elizabeth Poskitt in the UK, know that we appreciate the time they spent going through a draft of this book. Their comments resulted in many improvements.

We have received ideas, inspiration and help from many other people. These include: Marlou Bijlsma in Zimbabwe; Juliet Kayongo in Uganda; Anna Mswata, Biotshepo Giyose and Dr Saitoria in Tanzania; David Morley and Sally Grantham McGregor in the UK; Vicky Quinn in the USA and Sultana Khanum of the World Health Organization, Geneva. Darryl Cowley of TALC dealt with administrative details and Shirley Hamber, Sheila Jones and Linda Staniford of Macmillan Education nursed the manuscript into production.

Last but not least we are grateful to the following people and organisations for the illustrations: to David Gifford who made all the original drawings and modified Figures 7, 19 and 25; to Carol Aldous for Figures 12 and 21; to Felicity Savage for permission to use drawings from *Nutrition for developing countries* (Oxford University Press 1992) for Figures 9 and 27. Also we thank the World Health Organization for permission to use illustrations from *Training course on the management of severe malnutrition* (2002) for Figure 8; from *Management of the child with a serious infection or severe malnutrition* (2000) for Figure 15; and from *Complementary feeding: family foods for breastfed children* (2000) for Figure 26. Figures 7, 19 and 25 are modified WHO drawings. The photographs on the front cover (from the top clockwise) were kindly supplied by: Jean-Luc Ray/Aga Khan Foundation, Stephen Homewood, TALC courtesy of Felicity Savage and June Copeman (this image is also used for Figure 3) and Caroline Wilkinson. The photograph in Figure 5 was provided by Claire Schofield. We thank these people and organisations for permission to use their photographs.

Introduction

What the book is about

The book explains how to manage severely malnourished young children in hospitals or other health units with inpatient facilities. It describes the ten steps of treatment and highlights the role of mothers and other carers. It recognises HIV/AIDS as a common cause of malnutrition. We know that many health units are very short-staffed and often lack equipment and other resources. So, where possible, we suggest how to adapt procedures to these situations.

Who the book is for

Nurses, clinical officers, medical assistants and all other health workers, including doctors, responsible for malnourished children.

Other people who might use the book

Trainers and supervisors of health workers; those working in emergency situations.

Why we wrote the book

Many young children die from severe malnutrition because they receive inadequate care. In 1999, the World Health Organization published *Management of severe malnutrition* which gives well tested and updated guidelines for the treatment of children and adults. However this manual is mainly targeted at doctors. We discovered that many health workers wanted something that was simpler and easier to read. So we prepared this book and its accompanying CD Rom and website. These follow the WHO guidelines and are based on training modules for nurses developed at the University of the Western Cape, South Africa and the London School of Hygiene and Tropical Medicine, UK. The book will become part of this training package.

What the book does not cover

The book is short in order to keep the price low. So we have not included information on community care of malnourished children, the causes and prevention of malnutrition, the treatment of older children or adults or general ward management.

We hope that you will find the book easy to read and use. Please let us know if you have any comments about it. These will help us, and others, prepare better materials in future. In this way we can all contribute to improving the care of severely malnourished children.

Professor Ann Ashworth, London School of Hygiene and Tropical Medicine, UK
Ann Burgess, Nutrition Consultant, Scotland, UK

Explanation of words and terms

Apathy: not taking an interest in anything.
Catch-up growth: rapid weight gain that occurs when malnourished children are fed diets high in energy and protein to rebuild their lost tissues.
Cautious feeding: meeting energy and protein needs without stressing the liver, heart, kidneys or gut.
Chat: talk in an easy friendly way.
Cyanosis: bluish colour (lips, tongue, nails) due to slow blood flow.
Electrolytes: substances combined with sodium, potassium and magnesium that are dissolved in body fluids. They help maintain cell function and fluid balance.
Electrolyte imbalance: changes in the usual amounts of electrolytes in body fluids or in cells.
Hypoglycaemia: low blood glucose level.
Hypothermia: low body temperature.
Keratomalacia: condition of the cornea when it becomes cloudy and soft. The lens may come out.
Kwashiorkor: a severe form of malnutrition in which there is oedema of both feet.
Lethargy: lack of energy, not wanting to do anything.
Marasmic-kwashiorkor: a severe form of malnutrition in which there is both wasting and oedema.
Marasmus: a severe form of malnutrition in which there is extreme wasting.
Micronutrients: vitamins and minerals – nutrients needed in small (micro) amounts.
Motor development: movements that involve the legs and arms (e.g. crawling, walking) and more delicate movements (e.g. picking up and holding small objects).
Oedema: excess fluid in body tissues. In malnutrition, it is caused by electrolyte imbalances and nutrient deficiencies.
Oral Rehydration Salts Solution (ORS solution): solution containing sodium, potassium and glucose. Used to provide fluid in dehydration.
Pathogens: bacteria and viruses that cause disease. Sometimes called germs.
ReSoMal: **Re**hydration **So**lution for **Mal**nutrition. It provides less sodium than regular ORS solution and more potassium and glucose.
Severe malnutrition: condition where there is severe wasting and/or oedema.
Severe wasting: very thin; a weight-for-height of less than 70% of the normal weight-for-height.
Stunting: condition in which the child is too short.
Xerophthalmia: name given to eye signs caused by vitamin A deficiency.

1 Severely malnourished children need *different* care

> Severely malnourished children are *different* from other children.
> So they need *different* care.

Children become malnourished if they eat less than their bodies need to grow and be healthy. They may eat too little because there is not enough food at home or they are given too few meals. Sometimes their food is too watery and so is low in energy and nutrients. Sometimes no one encourages children to eat. Often they do not feel like eating because they are ill. Some children do not get enough breastmilk.

A few children become *severely* malnourished (see Figure 3 page 5 and Figure 5 page 6). This chapter explains how their bodies are *different* and why they need *different* care. The rest of the book describes how to look after these children.

The body of a severely malnourished child tries to keep the essential organs working by:

1 Reducing the amount of energy used. To do this the body may:
- Stop growing
- Decrease physical activity
- Reduce the work of some organs (e.g. the heart, liver and kidneys)
- Reduce activity inside cells (e.g. slowing the rate of pumping potassium in and sodium out)
- Decrease the body's response to infections (e.g. not producing a fever).

2 Using body fat and breaking down muscle and other tissues for energy.

Malnutrition causes visible changes

Appearance

Severely malnourished children:

- Are very thin and have loose skin (because they have lost fat and muscle)
- May have oedema (swelling) because of excess fluid
- May have skin and/or hair changes (because of cell damage).

Appetite

The children often have poor appetites. This may be due to infection and/or because their bodies are 'imbalanced' with too little of some nutrients and too much of others.

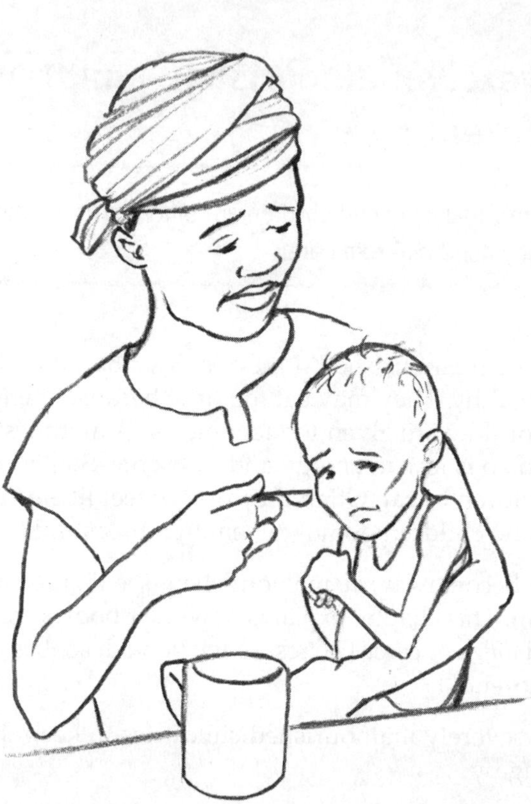

Figure 1 Severe malnutrition affects appearance, appetite and mood.

Mood

The children are often miserable, irritable and apathetic.

Malnutrition causes invisible (hidden) changes

We cannot see most of the changes because they affect organs and cells *inside* the body. Children may die if we ignore these changes or do not know about them when we treat these children.

Examples of invisible changes are:

- The liver cannot cope with large amounts of protein in the diet and also makes less glucose
- The heart becomes smaller and weaker. It cannot pump strongly and cannot deal with excess fluid in the blood
- The gut wall is thinner and makes fewer digestive enzymes. This decreases digestion and absorption of nutrients
- The kidneys cannot get rid of excess fluid or sodium

- The cell walls are 'leaky'. Potassium and magnesium leak out (and are excreted) and sodium leaks in. So the body contains too little potassium and magnesium and too much sodium. The excess sodium means that too much fluid stays in the body causing oedema
- The immune system is less efficient.

We explain these changes in more detail in Chapters 3–9.

Why severely malnourished children need *different* care

These children need *different* care from well nourished children because:

- Loss of muscle and a damaged liver increase the risk of hypoglycaemia
- Loss of body fat and low activity increase the risk of hypothermia
- The gut and liver cannot cope with normal meals
- The heart easily goes into heart failure if too much fluid is given
- Loss of fat and muscle makes it difficult to diagnose dehydration
- The inefficient immune system gives a weak response to infections so they may be missed.

This means that *severely* malnourished children must be:

- Fed differently from other children
- Rehydrated differently
- Treated with antibiotics even if there are no clinical signs of infection
- Given specific nutrients to correct electrolyte and fluid imbalances and repair damaged cells and organs
- Given special care (e.g. not kept waiting for admission, kept warm).

Without correct treatment the common causes of death in severe malnutrition are missed infection, heart failure, hypoglycaemia and hypothermia.

2 Assess the child

Severely malnourished children need priority care. Assess quickly and give any emergency treatment needed.

A nurse or other health worker should screen all children as they arrive at your hospital or health centre and identify those with severe malnutrition. Some may need emergency treatment. All other severely malnourished children must be seen quickly and not kept waiting.

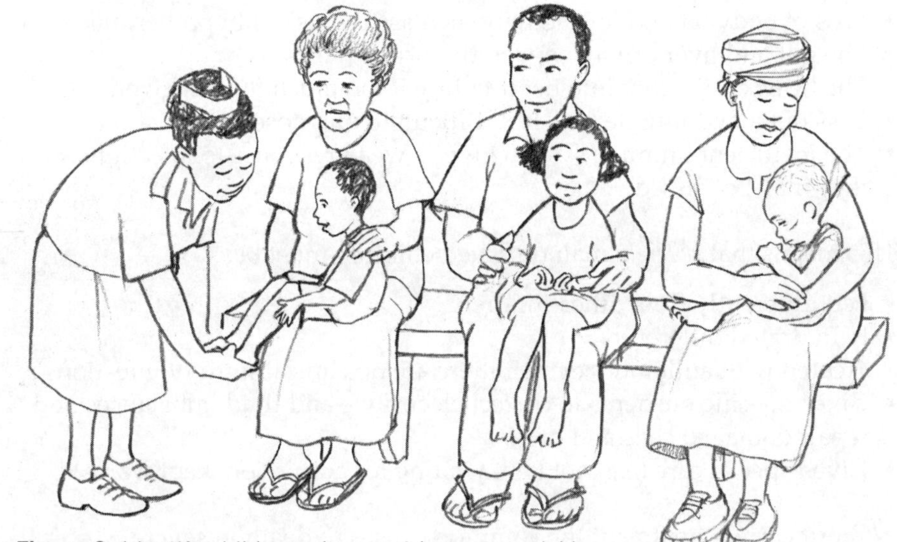

Figure 2 Identify children who must be seen quickly.

How to recognise severe malnutrition

A child has severe malnutrition if there is:

- Severe wasting *and/or*
- Oedema of both feet.

Recognising severe wasting

Severe wasting means extreme thinness. Look for wasting over the shoulders, ribs, upper arms, buttocks and thighs. The skin on the upper legs and buttocks may look like 'baggy pants'. The muscles may be so wasted that the child is too weak to walk or sit. The stomach may stick out ('pot belly') because the muscles are weak and there is gas in the upper gut. The face may look thin.

Wasted children are often anxious and irritable, and cry easily; sometimes they are quiet and apathetic. They may have a poor appetite but sometimes are very hungry.

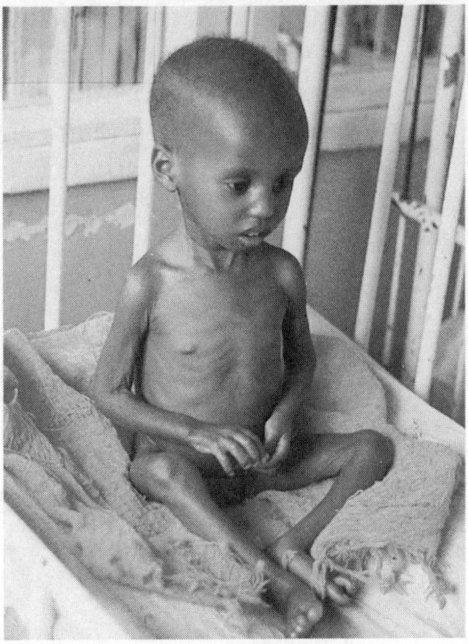

Figure 3 A child with severe wasting.

The weight is usually less than 60% of the healthy weight (in the red zone on some growth charts). However a low weight *may* be due to *stunting* and not wasting. Stunted children without wasting do *not* need hospital treatment.

You may see a recent drop in weight if the child has been weighed regularly.

Recognising oedema

Oedema usually occurs first in both feet and then in the lower legs. If the child has been lying down you may see oedema over the back. Oedema can quickly spread to the hands, lower arms and face. It may be mistaken for 'fatness'.

Table 2.1 classifies severity of oedema and Figure 4 shows how to test for oedema.

Table 2.1 *Classification of oedema*

Mild +	Feet only
Moderate ++	Feet, lower legs, hands, lower arms
Severe +++	Generalised oedema, including feet, legs, hands, arms and face

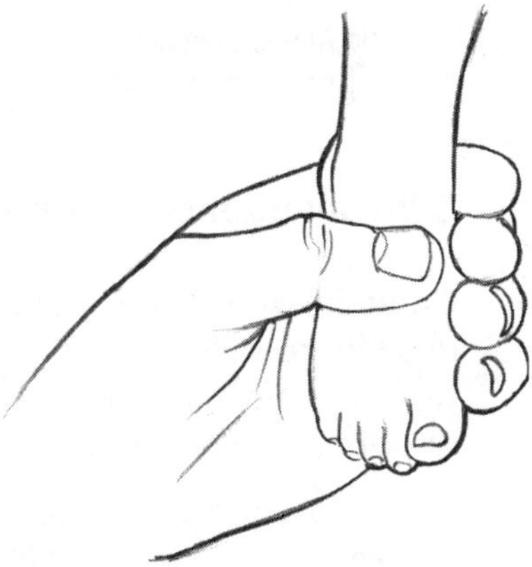

Figure 4 Test for oedema. *Hold both feet with your thumbs on top. Press gently for 10 seconds. Child has oedema if dents remain when you lift your thumbs.*

Malnourished children with oedema often have:

- Skin changes over swollen limbs and in the creases of the groin. Changes include abnormally dark, cracked, peeling patches ('flaky paint' dermatosis) with pale skin underneath that is easily damaged and infected

- Thin hair that can be easily pulled out. It may be paler and less curly than normal
- A poor appetite, and are miserable and apathetic.

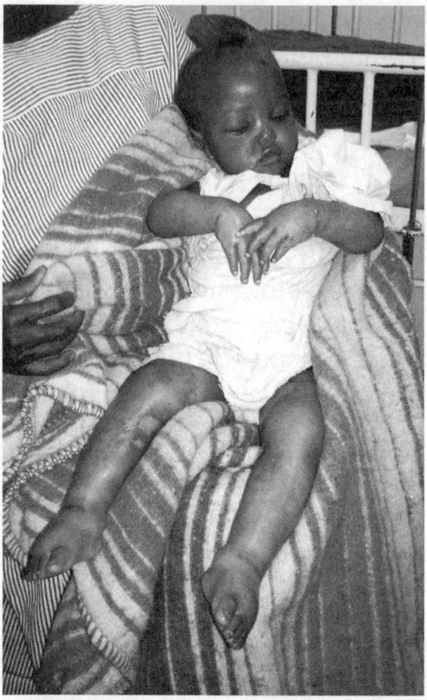

Figure 5 A child with severe oedema.

Box 2.1 ***Other terms for severe malnutrition***

Other terms are *marasmus* (severe wasting), *marasmic-kwashiorkor* (severe wasting + oedema) and *kwashiorkor* (oedema). We do not use the term 'protein–energy malnutrition' because malnutrition is usually the result of many nutrient deficiencies (including zinc and vitamin A) and infection.

Give emergency treatment

Children with severe malnutrition are very ill. So do the examination quickly, keeping the child covered as much as possible to avoid hypothermia. Give emergency treatment before taking a detailed history or doing a full examination or diagnostic tests:

- Give oxygen for severe respiratory distress
- Treat shock or severe dehydration. Treatment differs from standard treatment (see pages 20–21)
- Give emergency eye care if eyes have ulcers or look soft or cloudy (see Box 8.1 page 32)
- Arrange for a blood transfusion if the child is very breathless and there is severe pallor or the haemoglobin is less than 4 g/dl (see page 33)
- Treat hypoglycaemia (page 11) and hypothermia (page 14).

Take a history and do a full examination

The checklist in Box 2.2 may help you take a history and do a detailed examination. The diagnostic tests may help identify specific problems – they are not needed for successful treatment of malnutrition. A sample recording form is given in *Management of severe malnutrition* (see Appendix E page 77).

Box 2.2 ***Checklist for medical history and physical examination***

Collect only the information needed to guide treatment and advise the family. Do not ask all the questions at one time – choose an appropriate time and place for each question. Ask difficult questions (such as those about causes of deaths or drug abuse) only if really necessary and then ask in a culturally sensitive way.

Ask about feeding

- Foods and drinks taken in past few days
- Frequency of feeding
- Recent appetite
- Usual diet before ill
- When child last ate normally
- Breastfeeding history.

Ask about the medical history

- Vomiting and diarrhoea: duration and frequency; stools watery/bloody
- Thirst
- Time last passed urine
- Recent (within last few days) sinking of eyes
- Chronic cough
- Birth weight
- Birth rank
- Immunisations
- Milestones reached before ill (e.g. sitting, walking)
- Known or suspected HIV infection
- Recent contact with measles or tuberculosis.

Ask about the family

- Health problems and deaths of family members particularly the mother and siblings
- Social problems (e.g. drug and other abuse, teenage mother)
- Food security and living conditions (Severe malnutrition is often a sign that the family has problems).

Do physical examination

- Signs of shock
- Signs of pneumonia or heart failure
- Weight (and length or height if possible)
- Temperature, pulse and respiratory rates
- Face: puffy with swollen eyelids
- Eyes: signs of vitamin A deficiency (see Figure 14 page 31)
- Mouth: sore tongue, cracked lips, ulcers, thrush, throat infection
- Pallor of mouth, conjunctiva, palms (see Figure 15 page 33)
- Cyanosis: peripheral or central
- Jaundice
- Wasting: severity
- Oedema: severity
- Skin: peeling, lesions (infected, weeping)
- Enlarged glands
- Enlarged/tender liver.

►

Box 2.2 ***continued***

Do diagnostic tests
- Haemoglobin or packed cell volume
- Blood glucose (Dextrostix)
- Blood, urine, stool cultures if possible
- Malaria parasites
- Microscopy of urine (for infection) and of stools (for worms)
- Chest X-ray
- Skin test for TB. This may be falsely negative in malnourished children. Look for a BCG scar.

Routine treatment

Table 2.2 shows the ten steps for treating severe malnutrition and their approximate time frame. Chapters 3–12 explain how to carry out each step. Notice that although these are called 'steps' they do not happen one after the other. Most start on day 1.

Table 2.2 *Ten steps for treatment of severely malnourished children (approximate time frame)*

Step	*Action*	*Stabilisation*		*Rehabilitation*
		Days 1–2	*Days 3–7*	*Weeks 2–6*
1	Prevent or treat hypoglycaemia	••••••••••		
2	Prevent or treat hypothermia	••••••••••		
3	Prevent or treat dehydration	••••••••••		
4	Correct electrolyte imbalance	••••••••••	••••••••••	••••••••••
5	Treat and prevent infections	••••••••••	••••••••••	
6	Correct micronutrient deficiencies	•••No iron•••	••••••••••	With iron•••••
7	Start cautious feeding	••••••••••	••••••••••	
8	Give catch-up diet for rapid growth			•••••••••••••
9	Provide loving care, play and stimulation	••••••••••	••••••••••	••••••••••
10	Prepare for follow-up and discharge			•••••••••••••

The aim of the stabilisation phase is to:

- Treat infections and other urgent medical problems
- Provide sufficient energy and nutrients to stop further loss of muscle and fat
- Correct electrolyte imbalance

- Get rid of oedema
- Get the organs and cells working well again.

The aim of the rehabilitation phase is to:

- Provide extra energy and nutrients for rapid weight gain
- Give stimulating play to improve mental and motor development
- Make sure the carer and family know how to care for the child at home.

Use the checklist in Appendix D (pages 74–76) to monitor how well the ten steps are being carried out. Hold regular ward meetings to discuss the results and, if necessary, to plan how to improve performance.

Care for the carer

Mothers and other carers can do a lot to help their children recover. It is important to make them feel comfortable and to help them learn how to care for their children in hospital and when they go home. So, on admission:

- Make the mother or carer feel welcome – she (or he) is probably very scared and worried. Male carers may feel particularly anxious if most of the other carers are women. Have a male staff member talk with them
- Explain the ward routine and show the carer the toilets, washrooms and other facilities
- Tell the carer what she is expected to provide
- Introduce her to other carers and ask them to help her
- Make sure the carer knows she can ask questions and discuss problems with nurses and other staff.

When the carer has settled in arrange for a nurse or other health worker to talk confidentially with her. Make sure this person is very familiar with the treatment procedures, understands common local causes of malnutrition and knows how to counsel carers in a sympathetic way. The health worker should tell the carer:

- Why the child is sick and what treatment will be given (see pages 56–58)
- How long the child is likely to be in hospital
- That her care can help the child to recover more quickly.

If a carer knows the child is HIV+, tell her the child should improve with treatment but it may take longer than for other children.

3 Prevent or treat hypoglycaemia (Step 1)

Prevent hypoglycaemia by feeding malnourished children every 2–3 hours day and night. Start straightaway.

Hypoglycaemia means a low level of glucose in the blood (low blood sugar). Some of the food we eat is changed into glucose. The blood carries glucose to the cells that use it to produce energy.

Food → Glucose → Energy

Between meals, glucose normally comes from body stores or is made in the liver. Glucose is the main source of energy for the brain. The brain stops working properly if it does not get enough energy and the person may die.

Why malnourished children are at risk of hypoglycaemia

Severely malnourished children are likely to have low blood glucose because:

- They have poor appetites and so have less food to change to glucose
- The liver is damaged and makes less glucose than normal
- The muscles are wasted. Some glucose is stored in muscle. So children with wasted muscles have smaller stores of glucose
- They often have infections and need glucose to fight them. So they use glucose faster than normal
- They get cold easily and use glucose to try to keep warm.

Malnourished children *use glucose faster* than other children but they have *less glucose available.*

Malnourished children may develop hypoglycaemia if they:

- Have not been fed for several hours before admission (e.g. a child has diarrhoea so the carer does not give food; a child has a long wait before being admitted)
- Are not fed while being rehydrated
- Are not fed *at least* every 3 hours day and night
- Have an untreated infection
- Are cold.

How to diagnose hypoglycaemia

1 The best way to diagnose hypoglycaemia is to use a Dextrostix (Glucostix or glucose strip) preferably with a glucometer. A malnourished child is hypoglycaemic if the blood glucose level is below 3 millimoles per litre (<3 mmol/l). Use a level of below 4 mmol/l if there is no cut-off level at 3 mmol/l on the glucose strip. If you do not have a Dextrostix or cannot do the test immediately, assume the child is hypoglycaemic and treat (see below). It does no harm and may save the child's life.

2 Hypothermia is a sign of hypoglycaemia. The temperature falls if a child does not have enough glucose to keep warm. Check the temperature frequently (see page 13). If it is low (<35.5°C) assume the child is hypoglycaemic, and treat. Also warm the child. Hypoglycaemia and hypothermia often occur together and can be signs of serious infection (see pages 25–27 for treatment of infection).

3 A sign of *severe* hypoglycaemia is when an alert child becomes limp and drowsy (sleepy) and difficult to wake up. This can occur suddenly and is because too little glucose is getting to the brain. Watch for changes in mental state, particularly drowsiness. Ask carers to watch too.

How to prevent hypoglycaemia

Hypoglycaemia is most likely during the stabilisation phase and at night. To prevent:

- Feed starter formula *immediately* (see page 35)
- Feed every 3 hours day and night and at the correct times. Feed every 2 hours if the child is ill
- Keep the child warm to preserve glucose
- Start antibiotics immediately.

Tell the carer she can help by keeping the child warm and by feeding him frequently, especially at night.

How to treat hypoglycaemia

If the child is conscious:

1 Immediately give by mouth:
   - 50 ml of 10% glucose solution *or*
   - 50 ml starter formula *or*
   - 50 ml of 10% sugar solution. To make: dissolve 5 g (one rounded 5 ml teaspoon) sugar in 50 ml water.

   Give whichever is available quickest.

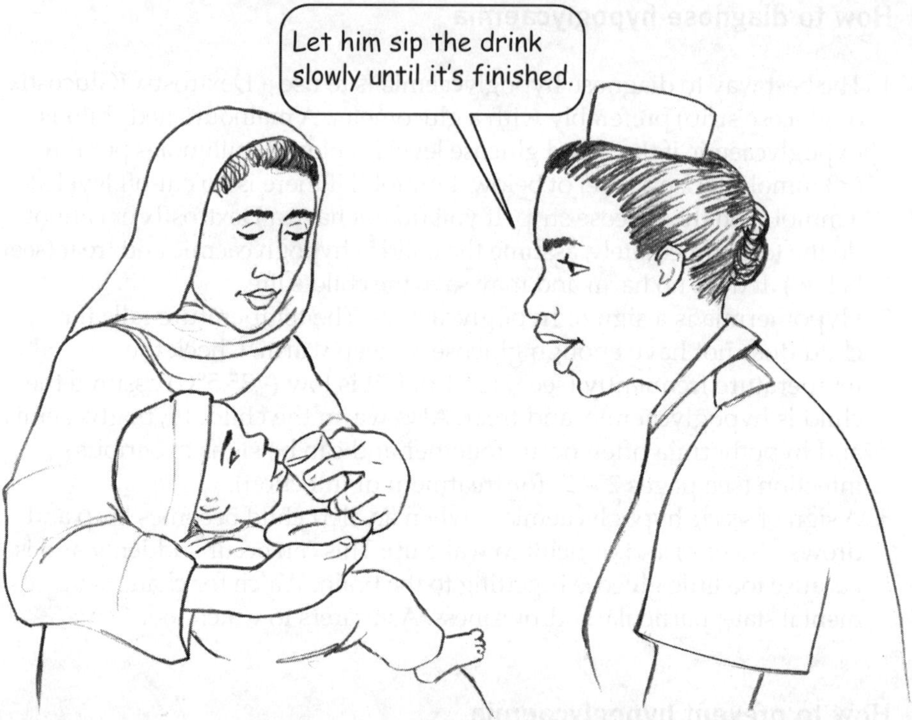

Figure 6 Feed immediately to prevent hypoglycaemia.

2 Begin starter formula within 30 minutes. Give every 2 hours for at least the first day.
3 Keep warm and start antibiotics immediately.

If the child is unconscious or convulsing:

1 Give glucose intravenously (IV) *immediately* (sterile 10% glucose solution 5 ml/kg body weight). If only 50% sterile dextrose solution is available dilute with sterile water (1 part sterile dextrose solution to 4 parts sterile water). If IV glucose cannot be given quickly, give 50 ml of 10% glucose solution or sugar solution by nasogastric tube.
2 Begin starter formula within 30 minutes. Give every 2 hours for at least the first day. Give by nasogastric tube if the child is not fully conscious.
3 Keep warm and start antibiotics immediately.

4 Prevent or treat hypothermia (Step 2)

Prevent hypothermia by keeping malnourished children warm and dry day and night and by feeding frequently.

Hypothermia means the body (rectal) temperature is below 35.5°C (95.9°F).

Why malnourished children are at risk of hypothermia

Severely malnourished children:

- Have lost fat so they have less protection from the cold
- Are less active than usual – activity produces heat
- Have been eating poorly. Food provides energy and heat
- Have less glucose available to use for energy and heat (see page 10).

Children are most likely to die from hypothermia:

- At night – because it is the coldest time and feeds might be missed due to carers sleeping or too few staff to supervise feeding
- In the first days after admission – because it takes time for the body to start working properly again and for antibiotics to cure infections.

How to diagnose hypothermia

The best way to diagnose hypothermia is to measure the temperature in the rectum. Use a low-reading thermometer or, if this is not available, an ordinary thermometer (blunt-ended if possible). Shake the mercury to below 35°C (or 95°F) and insert very carefully into the rectum to avoid internal damage. If the rectal temperature is below 35.5°C (95.9°F) or there is no reading on an ordinary thermometer the child has hypothermia.

A rectal temperature is better than an underarm temperature as it measures the temperature inside the body. If you must take the underarm temperature, leave the thermometer in place for at least 3 minutes. An underarm reading of below 35°C (95°F) means the child is too cold.

Monitor the temperature at least every 4 hours for the first few days. Also feel if the skin is cold with the back of your hand whenever you are near the child.

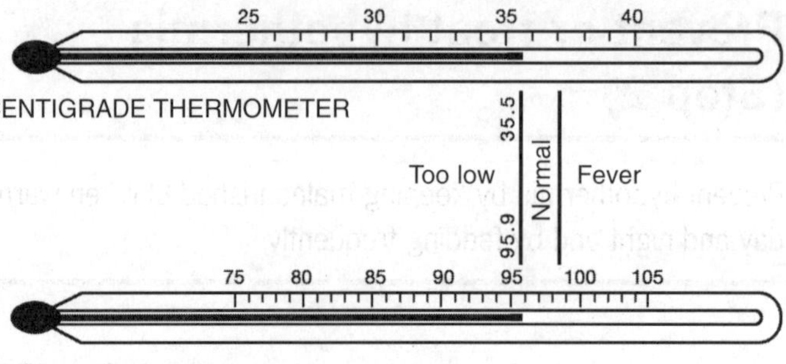

Figure 7 Cut-off temperature (rectal) for hypothermia.

How to prevent hypothermia

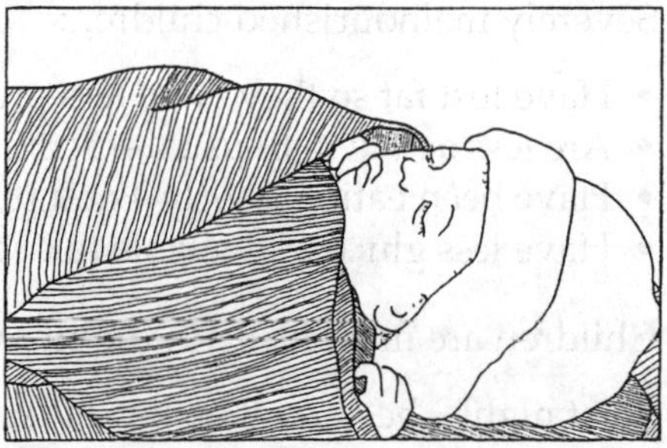

Figure 8 Dress the child warmly.

Severely malnourished children easily become too cold. To prevent hypothermia:

- Examine the child quickly and keep covered as much as possible
- Dress the child warmly, including the head, and cover with a blanket. Check the child is covered at night. Ask the carer to sleep with the child for warmth
- Keep the room hot. Use a heater if needed. Shut doors and windows and do not place the child near them
- Keep the child dry. Change wet clothes, nappies or bedding. Dry the child thoroughly after bathing. Do not bathe if very ill
- Feed frequently and at night
- Treat infections.

If the child has a high fever (42°C or above) sponge with slightly warm (not cold) water and check that the temperature does not fall too low.

How to treat hypothermia

1 Feed the child immediately and then every 2 hours for at least the first day.
2 Warm the child:
   - Dress in warm clothes, cover the head and wrap in a blanket. Place a heater or lamp nearby

- Or put in skin-to-skin contact with carer (kangaroo position) and cover both with a blanket.

If necessary, warm the clothes and bedding with a hot water bottle. Do *not* put a bottle near a child as it may damage the fragile skin – and bottles get cold quickly.

3 Monitor the temperature every 2 hours during rewarming (or every 30 minutes if using a heater). The temperature is normal when it is 36.5°C (98.4°F). Then keep the child warm but do not overheat.

Explain to the carer what you are doing. Tell her she can help by keeping the child warm and dry and feeding on time day and night.

5 Prevent or treat dehydration (Step 3)

> Too much fluid can kill. Rehydrate more slowly than usual. Do not give IV fluids except in shock.

Dehydration means having too little fluid in the body.

Why dehydration is difficult to diagnose in severe malnutrition

Table 5.1 (left side) shows the signs often used to diagnose dehydration in normal children. In severely malnourished children most of these may already be present (right side). This is because malnutrition can cause:

- Skin to lose its elasticity and eyes to become sunken due to loss of tissue
- Salivary glands to stop working.

If a malnourished child has a slow skin pinch (i.e. takes more than 2 seconds to flatten), sunken eyes or dry mouth, it is not possible to know if dehydration or malnutrition caused them. So it is difficult to diagnose dehydration in severely malnourished children.

It is also difficult to tell if a malnourished child is responding to treatment with rehydration fluid. The slow skin pinch, sunken eyes and dry mouth may remain even when the child is fully rehydrated. However it is important to look for these signs. If any go away when fluid is given, you know the child is being rehydrated.

Table 5.1 *Signs that occur in dehydration or severe malnutrition*

Usually present in dehydrated children	*Often present in severely malnourished children even when not dehydrated*
Skin pinch goes back slowly	Skin pinch goes back slowly
Sunken eyes	Sunken eyes
Dry mouth	Dry mouth
More thirsty than usual	

Tip: In malnourished children check for slow skin pinch over the breastbone where there is less loss of tissue.

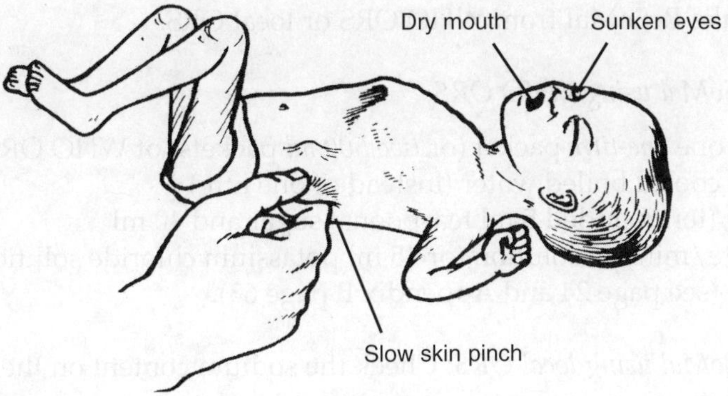

Figure 9 Do these signs tell if this malnourished child is dehydrated? *You cannot tell from these signs alone. More important signs are watery diarrhoea and more thirsty than usual.*

Deciding when to give rehydration fluid

Ask the carer if the child has watery diarrhoea. If the answer is yes, assume the child has some dehydration and treat. Malnourished children may pass many *small* unformed stools because their gut is damaged. These children do not need rehydration fluid. Children who vomit frequently may become dehydrated and need rehydration fluid. Children who have been vomiting before admission usually stop when fed small amounts of the starter formula.

Children with no diarrhoea or vomiting, who are drinking, are *not* dehydrated.

Danger of giving too much rehydration fluid

Severely malnourished children have weak hearts that cannot pump strongly. If too much fluid enters the blood they are likely to get heart failure and die. So always monitor for signs of fluid overload (see page 19) when giving rehydration fluid, and give it slowly and carefully.

How to treat dehydration

Severely malnourished children have too much sodium and too little potassium in their bodies (see page 22). Therefore use an oral rehydration fluid that contains *less* sodium and *more* potassium than regular (e.g. WHO) ORS solution. The rehydration fluid recommended is ReSoMal. This stands for **Re**hydration **So**lution for **Mal**nutrition. It has 45 mmol of sodium per litre, compared with 90 mmol in WHO ORS.

You can make ReSoMal from WHO ORS or local ORS.

To make ReSoMal using WHO ORS:

- Dissolve one *one-litre* packet (or *two 500 ml* packets) of WHO ORS in *2 litres* of cooled boiled water (instead of one litre)
- Add 50 g (ten rounded 5 ml teaspoons) sugar and 40 ml electrolyte/mineral solution (or 45 ml potassium chloride solution) if available (see page 24 and Appendix B page 63).

To make ReSoMal using local ORS: Check the sodium content on the label on the packet:

- If the label says that the ORS solution will contain 90 mmol sodium per litre use it to make ReSoMal as described above
- If the label says that the ORS solution will contain 60 mmol sodium per litre add 25 g (five rounded 5 ml teaspoons) sugar and 20 ml electrolyte/mineral solution (or 22.5 ml potassium chloride solution) to every *one litre* of solution.

WHO ORS and ReSoMal may be available from UNICEF (ask your UNICEF Country Office).

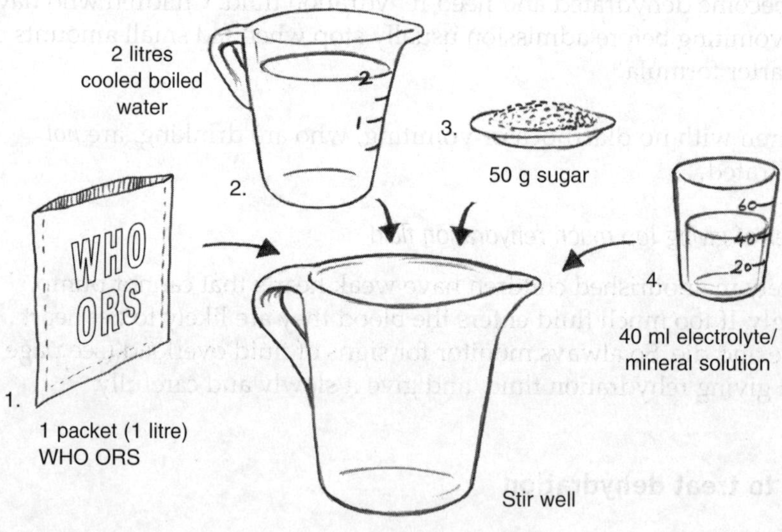

Figure 10 Preparing ReSoMal from WHO ORS packets.

Giving ReSoMal

- Rehydrate more slowly than you rehydrate well-nourished children. Give ReSoMal 5 ml/kg body weight every 30 minutes for the first

2 hours. Then give 5–10 ml/kg every hour for the next 4–10 hours. The exact amount and duration depends on how thirsty the child is and the size and frequency of the stools or vomit
- Show the mother how to give small sips slowly from a cup or spoon. Tell her it is important the child finishes the drink. If the child refuses to drink, tell her to be patient and keep trying. Give by nasogastric tube if the child cannot drink or is vomiting (see page 38)
- If the child is still receiving ReSoMal after 4 hours, give a feed of starter formula instead of ReSoMal. Then *continue* with ReSoMal each hour but *replace* with starter formula every 3 hours (or every 2 hours if the child is fed 2-hourly)
- Continue breastfeeding.

Do not give ReSoMal for more than 12 hours.

Monitor for signs of fluid overload

Record pulse and respiratory rates every 30 minutes for the first 2 hours when rehydrating a child. Then record every hour. *Stop* if there are signs of overload. These are:

- Increasing pulse rate (increase of 25 beats/minute or more) *and*
- Increasing respiratory rate (increase of 5 breaths/minute or more).

Another sign of fluid overload is increasing oedema (such as puffy eyelids) but increasing pulse and respiration rates are more important signs.

Signs of improvement are:

- Decreasing pulse and respiratory rates
- Less thirsty
- Passing urine
- Skin pinch is not as slow, eyes are less sunken and mouth is moist (although not all children show these changes)
- Child is more alert.

How to prevent dehydration in children with watery diarrhoea

If watery diarrhoea continues after the child is rehydrated, or if watery diarrhoea develops in hospital:

- Give 50–100 ml ReSoMal for each watery stool
- Give slowly from a cup or spoon; persuade the child to drink
- Continue feeding, including breastfeeding.

Emergency treatment of severe dehydration (shock)

Shock is a dangerous condition and requires emergency treatment. The common reasons for malnourished children to go into shock are severe dehydration and sepsis. Often both are present. It is not possible to find the cause of shock by examining the child. The only way is to see how the child responds to IV fluid. Children with dehydration respond to IV fluids. Those with septic shock do not and they quickly get fluid overload.

The signs of shock are:

- Child is lethargic or unconscious
- Cold hands (feel with the back of your hand)
- Capillary refill is longer than 3 seconds. To measure refill time, press on the nail to make it white and count the seconds until the pink colour returns
- A weak, fast pulse.

Treating shock

A child who has these four signs of shock must be kept warm and given:

- Oxygen
- IV glucose (5 ml/kg of 10% sterile glucose)
- IV fluids (see below)
- IV antibiotics (see page 25).

Explain to the carer what you are doing and why.

The best IV fluids for severely malnourished children are:

- Half-strength Darrow's with 5% dextrose *or*
- Ringer's lactate with 5% dextrose *or*
- 0.45% (half-normal) saline with 5% dextrose.

To start treatment:

- Give IV fluid 15 ml/kg over 1 hour. Use a paediatric giving set to prevent fluid entering too fast. Monitor the flow rate (drops/minute)
- Record pulse and respiration rates at the start and then *every 5–10 minutes* to check for fluid overload.

After 1 hour:

If there are signs of improvement (pulse and respiration rates are slower):

- Repeat IV 15 ml/kg over one more hour. Do not rehydrate with IV fluids for more than 2 hours

- Then change to oral or nasogastric rehydration with ReSoMal 10 ml/kg per hour for up to 10 hours
- After 4 hours, replace ReSoMal with starter formula (if the child is still receiving ReSoMal) and then give starter formula whenever a feed is due.

If there is no improvement after one hour assume the child has septic shock:

- Give maintenance fluids (4 ml/kg per hour)
- Transfuse with fresh whole blood 10 ml/kg *slowly* over 3 hours; give furosemide first (1 mg/kg IV).

If the child gets worse during treatment, stop IV fluids.

6 Correct electrolyte imbalance (Step 4)

> Electrolyte imbalance can cause heart failure. To correct electrolyte imbalance, give extra potassium and magnesium daily. Limit sodium (salt).

Three electrolytes are important in malnutrition: potassium, magnesium and sodium. In a healthy body, most of the potassium and magnesium is inside the cells and most sodium is outside the cells. This arrangement is needed for correct fluid balance and for cells to work properly. In severe malnutrition the body loses potassium and magnesium and builds up sodium.

How electrolyte imbalance develops

Malnourished children's bodies have too little potassium and magnesium because:

- Potassium and magnesium leak out of the cells and are excreted in urine. They leak out because malnutrition damages cell walls. Lack of micronutrients means the cell walls cannot be repaired. Also the tiny pumps in the cell wall (that should keep potassium and magnesium in and sodium out) work slowly to save energy
- Potassium and magnesium are lost during diarrhoea and when muscle is broken down to make essential energy
- Intakes of potassium and magnesium have been low because children have eaten too little food.

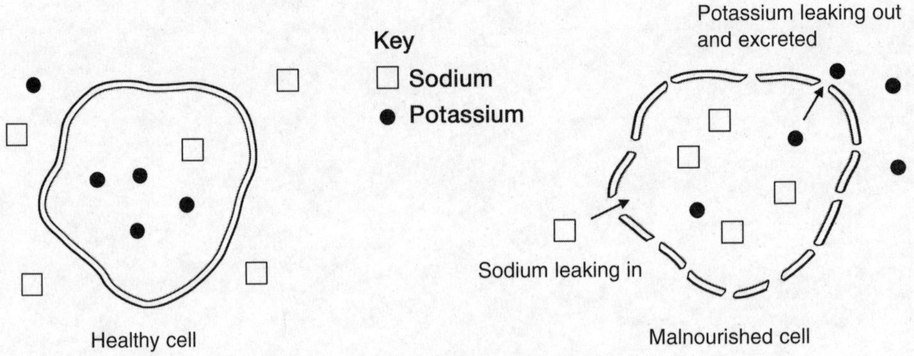

Figure 11 Diagrams of a healthy cell and a malnourished cell. *The malnourished cell has too much sodium and has lost potassium.*

Their bodies have too much sodium and are 'too salty' because:

- The damaged kidneys do not excrete excess sodium
- Sodium leaks into the cells through the damaged cell walls and the tiny pumps are working slowly.

Why electrolyte imbalance matters

Excess sodium 'pulls' extra water into the spaces between the cells and causes oedema. Too much fluid in the body increases the risk of heart failure. Loss of potassium weakens the heart so also increases the risk of heart failure. A child with electrolyte imbalance feels apathetic and weak and has a poor appetite.

Correcting electrolyte imbalance helps to get rid of oedema, prevent heart failure, make the cells work normally and improve appetite. Giving potassium and magnesium also helps to rebuild tissues.

How to treat electrolyte imbalance

Diagnosis

Most changes due to electrolyte imbalance take place inside cells so we cannot see them. The main visible sign of electrolyte imbalance is oedema. Other signs are a poor appetite and apathy. But *all* severely malnourished children have electrolyte imbalance, so all need treatment.

Measuring electrolytes in blood is likely to give the *wrong* diagnosis. The sodium level is likely to be low (even though the body is too salty) because much has leaked from the blood into the cells. The potassium level may seem normal because much has leaked from the cells into the blood.

Treatment

1 Give extra potassium and magnesium daily for at least 2 weeks.
2 Use ReSoMal for treating dehydration and low-sodium IV fluids for treating shock.
3 Do not add salt or flavouring cubes when cooking children's food; do not add salt to cooked food. Tell carers that children must not have salty food – so carers should not share their meals or snacks.

Do not treat oedema with diuretics. It increases the loss of potassium and makes electrolyte imbalance worse.

Potassium is *essential* for recovery. Give extra potassium (4 mmol/kg per day) as:

- Electrolyte/mineral solution (see recipe in Appendix B page 63). Give 20 ml in each one litre of starter formula, catch-up formula and ReSoMal *or*
- 10% stock potassium chloride solution (100 g KCl in one litre water). Give 22.5 ml in each one litre of starter formula, catch-up formula and ReSoMal *or*
- Slow K. Give $\frac{1}{2}$ crushed tablet/kg per day. (K is the symbol for potassium.)

Give extra magnesium (0.6 mmol/kg per day) as:

- Electrolyte/mineral solution (see above) *or*
- 2% magnesium sulphate solution. Give 1 ml with food 3–4 times a day *or*
- 50% magnesium sulphate solution. Give 0.3 ml/kg intramuscularly once to a maximum of 2 ml.

7 Treat and prevent infections (Step 5)

> Give broad-spectrum antibiotics to *all* severely malnourished children to prevent death from hidden infections. Wash hands to prevent cross-infection.

Infections are common in severely malnourished children. But signs used to diagnose infection (e.g. fever, increased pulse and respiration rates, redness) are often absent because children have damaged immune systems. This means that even very serious infections such as septicaemia can be missed.

Preventing death from hidden infections

Assume all severely malnourished children have hidden infections and treat with antibiotics (see Table 7.1). Do not wait for laboratory results as

Table 7.1 *Antibiotics recommended for severely malnourished children*

If:	*Give:*
No complications	Co-trimoxazole oral 5 ml (240 mg) every 12 hours for 5 days (2.5 ml (120 mg) if child weighs less than 6 kg) **Plus** metronidazole oral (7.5 mg/kg) every 8 hours for 7 days
Complications (shock, hypoglycaemia, hypothermia, dermatosis with skin lesions, respiratory or urinary tract infections, or lethargic/sickly appearance)	Gentamicin* IV or IM (7.5 mg/kg), once daily for 7 days **Plus** metronidazole oral (7.5 mg/kg) every 8 hours for 7 days **Plus** ampicillin IV or IM (50 mg/kg), every 6 hours for 2 days **followed by**: amoxicillin† oral (15 mg/kg), every 8 hours for 5 days
If child fails to improve within 48 hours, **Add**:	Chloramphenicol IV or IM (25 mg/kg), every 8 hours for 5 days. (Give every 6 hours if you suspect meningitis)

* If the child is not passing urine, gentamicin may accumulate in the body and cause deafness. Do not give the second dose until the child is passing urine.

† If amoxicillin is not available, give ampicillin, 50 mg/kg orally every 6 hours for 5 days.

Table 7.2 *Doses for specific formulations and body weights*

Antibiotic	*Route/Dose/ Frequency/Duration*	*Formulation*	*Dose according to child's weight*		
			3 kg up to 6 kg	*6 kg up to 8 kg*	*8 kg up to 10 kg*
Amoxicillin	Oral: 15 mg/kg every 8 hours for 5 days	Tablet, 250 mg	¼ tablet	½ tablet	½ tablet
		Syrup, 125 mg/5 ml	2.5 ml	5 ml	5 ml
		Syrup, 250 mg/5 ml	1.5 ml	2 ml	2.5 ml
Ampicillin	Oral: 50 mg/kg every 6 hours for 5 days	Tablet, 250 mg	1 tablet	1½ tablets	2 tablets
	IV/IM: 50 mg/kg every 6 hours for 2 days	Vial of 500 mg mixed with 2.1 ml sterile water to give 500 mg/2.5 ml	1 ml	1.75 ml	2.25 ml
Metronidazole	Oral: 7.5 mg/kg every 8 hours for 7 days	Suspension, 200 mg/5 ml	1 ml	1.25 ml	1.5 ml

the child may get worse if treatment is delayed. Medicines can be modified later if necessary. Give children who look ill or have complications:

- IV/IM antibiotics. They work faster
- Gentamicin, or other antibiotic that works against Gram-negative bacteria, to prevent septicaemia.

Hypoglycaemia and hypothermia are danger signs of serious infection. Severely malnourished children with infection are more likely to have a low temperature than fever.

Treatment

Give broad-spectrum antibiotics. Tables 7.1 and 7.2 show the recommended schedule and dosages. If some antibiotics are unavailable, follow your hospital's policy for broad-spectrum antibiotic treatment in children, including Gram-negative cover. Make sure you give the correct amount on time and that the child completes the course. Antibiotics only work effectively if there is a constant level in the body.

Table 7.2 shows the doses for children of different weights. For chloramphenicol calculate the *exact* dose using the child's weight.

Care for skin lesions (dermatosis) so they do not become infected:

- Keep lesions dry. Cover with a dry dressing to keep them clean and free of flies
- Stop skin oozing and itching by soaking in 0.01% potassium permanganate or dab with gentian violet. Put zinc and castor oil ointment, petroleum jelly or paraffin gauze on raw areas
- If the child is scratching, put mittens on or bandage the hands
- Remove nappies if the bottom or groin is sore.

Follow local guidelines for treating malaria if there is a positive blood slide, or if malaria is suspected.

How to prevent infections in the ward

Severely malnourished children have poor immunity and easily catch new infections in hospital. Figure 12 shows how children may get an infection from other people. Show carers how they can help protect their children from infection (see page 58).

Preventing person-to-person infection

Staff should wash hands *before* touching each child and *after* using the toilet or changing soiled nappies, clothes, bed linen, etc. There should be

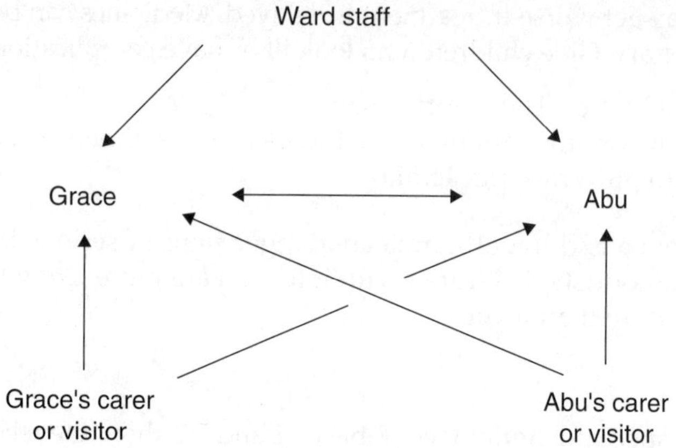

Figure 12 How infections can spread.

hand-washing facilities with soap in each ward and in all toilets (for staff, carers and patients). Staff and carers should handle soiled nappies, clothes, etc. carefully and keep flies off them. Ask them to put these items in fly-proof bins or sealed plastic bags if possible. Other ways to prevent infections are by:

- Disinfecting thermometers each time after use
- Giving measles vaccine to children on admission (if aged 6 months or older and not already vaccinated).

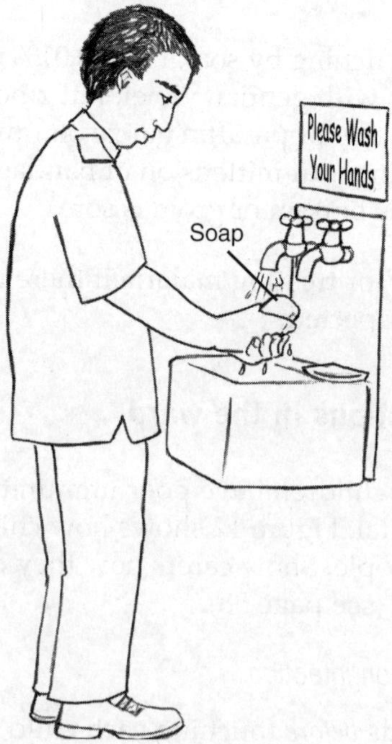

Figure 13 Wash hands thoroughly with soap to prevent infections spreading.

Many malnourished children and carers are HIV+ but you may not know their HIV status. So take precautions when nursing all malnourished children (e.g. use needles only once).

Preventing infections through skin

- Avoid unnecessary punctures
- Care for broken skin (see above)
- Keep clothes and bedding dry.

Preventing infections through water and food

Staff and carers should wash hands before preparing feeds or feeding children. Feeding utensils should be sterilised or cleaned with soap. Do not use them for more than one child without washing. Sterilise nasogastric tubes and keep in a clean place. Staff should also:

- Prepare feeds and ReSoMal with boiled water
- Use cups and spoons for feeding, never bottles
- Keep feeds and other food covered and stored in a refrigerator if possible
- Keep kitchen and ward clean and free from pests such as flies, cockroaches and rats.

8 Correct micronutrient deficiencies (Step 6)

To correct micronutrient deficiencies give extra vitamin A, zinc, copper, folic acid and multivitamins. Do not give iron at first; wait until the child has started the rehabilitation phase.

Why severely malnourished children need extra micronutrients

Malnourished children lack micronutrients. Common reasons are:

- An inadequate home diet
- Some micronutrients (e.g. zinc) are lost in stools during diarrhoea
- Their bodies have used micronutrients to fight infections.

Effect of micronutrient deficiencies

Table 8.1 shows that lack of micronutrients causes or worsens some conditions.

Table 8.1 *Effect of micronutrient deficiencies*

Deficiency of:	*Is associated with:*
Vitamin A	Changes in the eyes (see Figure 14) and blindness Weak immune system Increased risk of severe infection Increased risk of dying
Multiple micronutrients	Cell damage (leaky cells, oedema, skin and hair changes)
Zinc, folic acid	Damaged gut; diarrhoea
Zinc, multiple micronutrients	Cracked peeling skin; poor appetite
Iron, folic acid, vitamin A	Anaemia
B vitamins	Cracks at corners of mouth; smoother or sore tongue

Give extra micronutrients to:

- Prevent blindness
- Repair the immune system
- Repair cells and get rid of oedema

- Repair the damaged gut and stop diarrhoea
- Heal the skin
- Improve appetite
- Rebuild muscle and other cells.

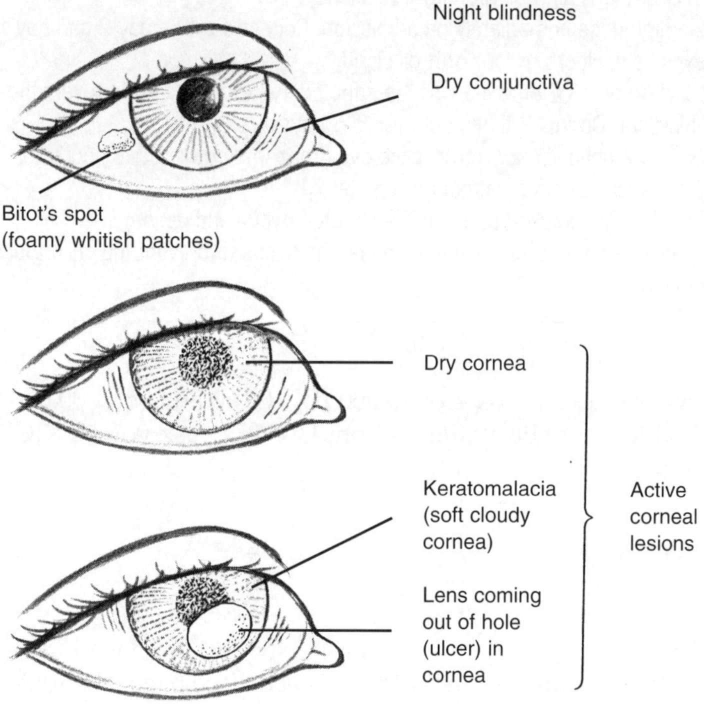

Figure 14 Eye signs of vitamin A deficiency (xerophthalmia).

How to correct micronutrient deficiencies

Vitamin A

Most severely malnourished children lack vitamin A, even if they have no eye signs (see Figure 14). They are at risk of developing xerophthalmia. Give one high dose of vitamin A on admission (day 1). Do not give if you are sure the child has received a high dose in the previous month. Check the dosage of the capsules and give:

- 50,000 IU if age is less than 6 months
- 100,000 IU if age is 6–12 months
- 200,000 IU if age is over 12 months.

Give further treatment if there is any sign of xerophthalmia (see Box 8.1) as children can go blind very quickly – within hours.

Box 8.1 ***How to treat xerophthalmia***

Children with xerophthalmia may not want to open their eyes. Examine them *very* gently to prevent breaking the cornea. If the cornea breaks, the lens can push out and cause blindness.

If a child has any eye sign of vitamin A deficiency:

1 Give one high dose immediately on admission. Repeat dose on day 2 and day 14.
2 If the eyes have ulcers or look soft or cloudy:
  - Put 1 drop of 0.1% atropine into the affected eye to relax it and prevent the lens pushing out. Do this 3 times daily for 3–5 days
  - Instil chloramphenicol or tetracycline eye drops (as required 2–3 hourly for 7–10 days). Never use ointment containing steroids
  - Put 0.9% saline soaked pads on the affected eye(s) and bandage
  - If necessary put mittens or bandages on the hands to prevent the child touching the eyes.

Vitamin A capsules (in doses of 10,000 IU, 100,000 IU and 200,000 IU) and folic acid tablets may be available from UNICEF (ask your UNICEF Country Office).

Other micronutrients

Give:

- Zinc (2 mg/kg per day) and copper (0.3 mg/kg per day). Give as electrolyte/mineral solution added to feeds (see page 24 and Appendix B pages 63–66). If this solution is not available give 1 ml/kg per day of 1.5% zinc acetate solution (15 g in one litre water)
- 2.5 mg folic acid daily
- 5 ml multivitamin syrup daily.

Do *not* give iron during the stabilisation phase.

Why iron is not given at first

Anaemia is common in malnourished children but giving iron too early is dangerous. This is because the blood may have too little protein to hold on to (bind) the iron and keep it safe. Unbound iron can:

- Damage cell walls and make them leaky
- Stimulate the growth of some harmful bacteria and makes infections worse.

So start iron supplements in the rehabilitation phase when there has been time for iron to be bound and antibiotics to kill harmful bacteria.

Box 8.2 ***Iron***

When the child enters the rehabilitation phase give iron 3 mg/kg per day. Give twice a day between meals by mouth – never by injection. If the child is anaemic (haemoglobin <11 g/dl and/or has pallor of the palms) continue treatment at home for 3 months.

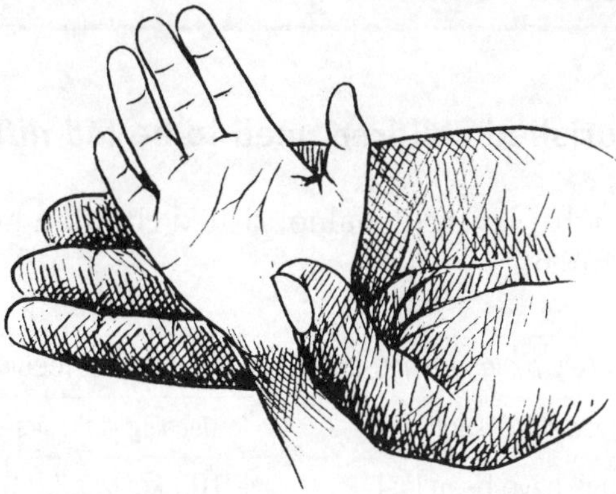

Figure 15 Examine for pallor of the palms. *Compare the colour of the child's palm to that of a healthy person.*

Treatment of severe anaemia

Anaemia is only a serious problem if it is very severe and there is a risk of heart failure. Severe pallor is a sign of severe anaemia. A child urgently needs a *very carefully* administered small blood transfusion (10 ml/kg of whole fresh blood slowly over 3 hours) if:

- Haemoglobin is below 4 g/dl (or below 3 g/dl if blood for transfusion is not screened for HIV and hepatitis)
- Haemoglobin is 4–6 g/dl and the child is breathless and has a weak, rapid pulse.

Give furosemide (1 mg/kg IV) at the start of the transfusion to make space for the blood, by reducing the amount of fluid in the bloodstream.

9 Start cautious feeding (Step 7)

Give small amounts of starter formula every 2–3 hours day and night. Starter formula is specially designed to meet the needs of severely malnourished children.

Severely malnourished children need to be fed *differently*

Table 9.1 explains why severely malnourished children need special feeds at the start of treatment.

Table 9.1 *Why severely malnourished children need different feeding*

Organ/tissue	*Changes in malnutrition*	*So for feeding in the first few days:*
Fat and muscle	Tissues have been lost	Give 100 kcal/kg body weight per day. This will stop further tissue loss
Liver	Cannot cope with lots of protein. Makes less glucose	Give 1 g protein/kg body weight per day. This is enough to cover basic needs Give sugary feed to provide glucose
Heart	Is small and weak and cannot cope with excess fluid	Measure feed intake Give 130 ml/kg body weight per day Give 100 ml/kg body weight per day if child has *severe oedema*
Kidneys	Cannot get rid of excess fluid or sodium	Measure feed intake Restrict sodium
Gut	Has less enzymes. Has less surface for absorbing nutrients	Give small, frequent feeds. Small feeds reduce the risk of diarrhoea. Frequent feeds prevent hypoglycaemia and hypothermia

So feed severely malnourished children:

- A special 'starter formula' for the first few days. Starter formula is low in protein and sodium and high in sugar
- Small amounts every 3 hours day and night (8 feeds over 24 hours). Feed very ill children every 2 hours if possible (12 feeds over 24 hours).

Starter formula

Ingredients

Starter formula must contain milk, sugar and oil:

- Milk is essential. It is important to obtain it even if it is expensive. About 200 ml fresh milk or 25 g full cream milk powder makes enough starter formula for a 5 kg child for a day
- Sugar provides the glucose needed to prevent hypoglycaemia. It makes the formula taste very sweet
- Oil provides extra energy in a small volume.

Appendix B pages 63–65 lists the ingredients and methods for making 1000 ml (one litre) of starter formula. Each recipe provides 75 kcal and 0.9 g protein per 100 ml. Starter formula is called F-75 in some publications.

How much to feed

- If the child has no oedema (or only mild or moderate oedema) give 130 ml starter formula/kg body weight per day. This provides 100 kcal and 1 g protein/kg body weight per day. It is enough to cover basic needs without overloading the child's weak body
- If a child has *severe oedema* (see Table 2.1 page 5) give *100 ml*/kg body weight per day.

Chart 1 in Appendix C pages 70–71 shows the volumes of feed needed by children of different weights and oedema status (see examples below). This provides the right amount of fluid, energy and protein at the start of treatment. Keep the amount the same for the next few days even if the child gains or loses weight. It will be increased in the rehabilitation phase. Note that Chart 1 is in two parts. Use the left side for children with no oedema (or only mild or moderate oedema). Use the right side for children with severe oedema.

Examples of calculating the amount for each 3-hourly feed

Method A using Chart 1

Kofi weighed 5.4 kg on admission and had no oedema. Chart 1 shows that he needs 90 ml at each 3-hourly feed.

Grace weighed 7.8 kg on admission and had severe oedema. Chart 1 shows that she needs 100 ml at each 3-hourly feed.

Method B

Kofi weighed 5.4 kg on admission and had no oedema. Amount of formula needed for 24 hours = 130 ml x 5.4 kg = 702 ml. So amount needed at each of the eight 3-hourly feeds = 702 ml/8 = 88 ml (or 90 ml).

Grace weighed 7.8 kg on admission and had severe oedema. Amount of formula needed for 24 hours = 100 ml x 7.8 kg = 780 ml. So amount needed at each of the eight 3-hourly feeds = 780 ml/8 = 98 ml (or 100 ml).

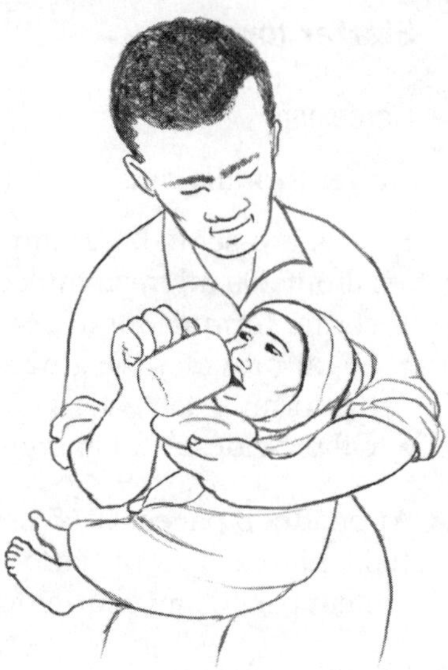

Figure 16 How to feed correctly.

To calculate the amount of each feed for a child needing twelve 2-hourly feeds:

1 Find the total amount needed for 24 hours by multiplying the child's admission weight by 130 ml. (Multiply the admission weight by 100 ml if the child has severe oedema).
2 Divide this amount by 12.

Or use Chart 1 and multiply the 3-hourly amount by 8. Then divide this amount by 12.

Examples of calculating the amount for each 2-hourly feed

Thandi weighed 3.4 kg on admission and had hypoglycaemia but no oedema. She was prescribed 2-hourly feeds. Amount of formula needed for 24 hours = 130 ml x 3.4 kg = 442 ml. So amount needed at each of the 12 2-hourly feeds = 442 ml/12 = 37 ml (or 40 ml).

Kim weighed 8.2 kg on admission and had severe oedema. He looked very ill and was prescribed 2-hourly feeds. So amount of formula needed for 24 hours = 100 ml x 8.2 kg = 820 ml. So the amount needed at each of the 12 2-hourly feeds = 820 ml/12 = 68 ml (or 70 ml).

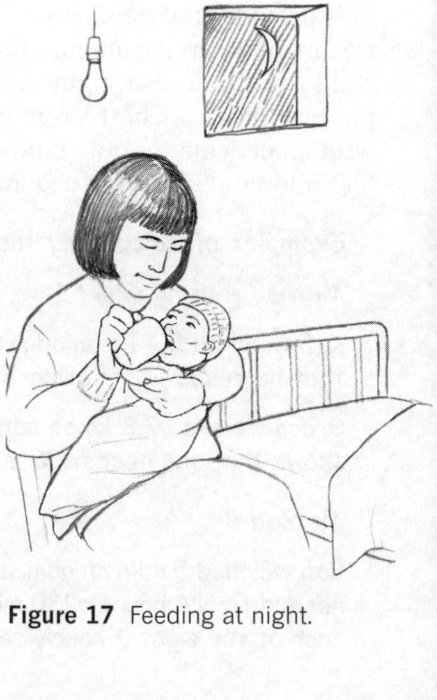

Figure 17 Feeding at night.

How to feed

- Give the feed by cup or small spoon. Never use bottles as they are easily contaminated. Sit the child on the carer's lap (never feed lying down). Show the carer how to hold a saucer under the child's chin to catch spills and dribbles (see Figure 16)

- Show the carer how to feed in small sips especially if the child is anorexic. Tell her to be patient. It may take a long time to give all the feed but it is one of most important ways she can help the child
- If the child vomits, wait 10 minutes and then offer the feed again. If the child vomits again, give the sips more slowly. Ask the carer to tell you if the child vomits
- Supervise carers especially at night so that feeds are not missed or given late. Explain to carers that feeding frequently at night may be a nuisance but can save the child's life. As soon as the child is better they will not need to wake up so often.

Breastfeeding

Malnutrition in a breastfed child is a sign that breastfeeding has been inadequate. Breastfeeding cannot be relied upon for treatment. So give all breastfed children the prescribed amounts of starter formula. Encourage children to breastfeed after finishing the formula. This improves the mother's milk supply so she can breastfeed successfully at home.

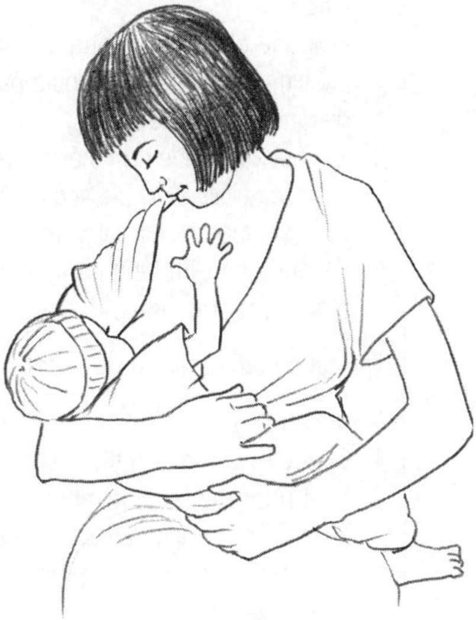

Figure 18 Breastfeed after giving starter formula.

If the child is too weak to breastfeed, show the mother how to express her milk. If breastfeeding has stopped and the child is under 6 months, encourage the mother to re-establish her milk supply (for details see *Relactation: review of experience and recommendations for practice* in Appendix E page 78).

Nasogastric feeding

Children will get worse and may die if they do not get enough starter formula. Feed by nasogastric tube if a child:

- Is lethargic and refuses to eat
- Has refused or vomited the last two consecutive feeds
- Has taken less than the minimum amount needed over the past 24 hours (see Chart 1 page 70).

Example

Grace weighed 7.8 kg on admission and had severe oedema. She was prescribed 100 ml starter formula at each 3-hourly feed. On day 2 she only took a total of 310 ml (see Chart 3 page 73). This is less than the 620 ml cut-off for a 7.8 kg child with severe oedema (see Chart 1 page 71). So Grace was tube fed on day 3.

Box 9.1 ***How to give a nasogastric feed***

Nasogastric feeding must be done by experienced staff. Before you start explain to the carer what you are doing and why.

How to insert a nasogastric tube

1 Use tube size 8 French.
2 Figure 19 shows how to measure the length of tubing to insert. Mark the tube at this length.
3 Hold the child firmly, lubricate the tip of the tube with water and pass into one nostril, pushing it slowly in. It should pass easily into the stomach. Stop when the measured distance is reached.
4 To check the tube is in the stomach, fill a syringe with air and listen with stethoscope over stomach while air is pushed down the tube from the syringe. If the tube is in the stomach you can hear the air entering the stomach.
5 Fix the tube with tape firmly to the nose so it cannot move during feeding or if the child touches it or coughs.

The tube can remain in place for several days.

How to feed

1 Check the tube is in the stomach (see above).
2 First offer the feed by mouth.
3 Fix a 20-ml syringe (without plunger) to the end of the tube.
4 Then pour the remaining feed into the syringe and let it flow in by gravity. Do not press in by plunger.

Monitor progress

To monitor the progress of each child:

1 Record (using Chart 3 page 73):
   - The amounts of feed offered, left over and/or vomited so you know how much was eaten and not vomited
   - Episodes of watery diarrhoea.
2 Weigh and plot the weight each day (see Figure 21 page 43). Children on starter formula should maintain their weight unless they have oedema – then they should lose weight.

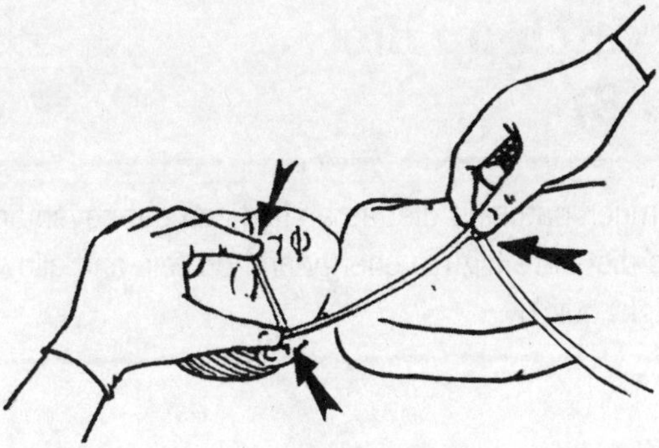

Figure 19 Measuring a nasogastric tube. *Measure the distance from the nose to the ear and then to the xiphisternum (base of the breastbone). Insert the tube to this measured distance.*

10 Give catch-up diet (Step 8)

Give as much catch-up diet as a child can eat seven times a day. Catch-up diets are high in energy and protein and allow the child to gain weight quickly.

Children enter the rehabilitation phase when infections are under control and their bodies are beginning to work properly again. Signs that a child has reached this phase are when he becomes very hungry and easily finishes his feed, and most or all of his oedema has gone. Usually the child starts to smile and becomes more active.

Changing to a catch-up diet

It is important to change to a catch-up diet as soon as children are ready, as starter formula does not contain enough energy and protein for rapid weight gain. Most children are ready for a catch-up diet 3–4 days after admission. Some are ready in 1–2 days. Very ill children or those with severe oedema may take about a week.

Changing from starter formula to catch-up formula

At the beginning of the rehabilitation phase children are very hungry. If they are allowed to eat unlimited amounts of catch-up diet immediately they may suddenly develop heart failure. So restrict intake for the first 3 days like this:

1. On the first two days (transition day 1 and 2) replace starter formula with the same volume of catch-up formula and feed 3-hourly day and night.
2. On the third day (transition day 3) increase each feed by 10 ml until the child leaves some. Feed 3-hourly day and night.

After the 3 transition days:

- Feed as much as the child wants and breastfeed often. A carer should ask for more food if her child finishes his feed
- Feed at least seven times each day. For example, feed 3-hourly but leave out one night feed
- Continue to give extra electrolytes and micronutrients
- Start iron (see Box 8.2 page 33).

Catch-up diets

What to feed

Give a milk-based catch-up formula at the beginning of the rehabilitation phase and to children aged under 6 months. For older children gradually replace the catch-up formula by diets based on enriched porridges or other family foods. Catch-up diets are high in energy, protein and some micronutrients. This allows children to build new fat and muscle quickly and regain weight.

Appendix B pages 65–66 lists the ingredients and methods for making 1000 ml (one litre) of milk-based catch-up formula. Each recipe contains 100 kcal and 3 g protein per 100 ml. In some publications catch-up formula is called F-100. It contains more milk and oil and less sugar than starter formula. If milk is scarce, make catch-up diets from staple foods (e.g. thick cereal porridge) and add:

- A fat-rich food (e.g. oil or margarine) to make sure the diet contains enough energy *and*
- Pea, bean, groundnut, soya or other oilseed flours/pastes, fish powder or eggs for extra protein. Oilseed flours and pastes (e.g. peanut butter) provide energy *and* protein so are useful for enriching meals.

Give high energy snacks such as bread and margarine between feeds. Avoid salty foods.

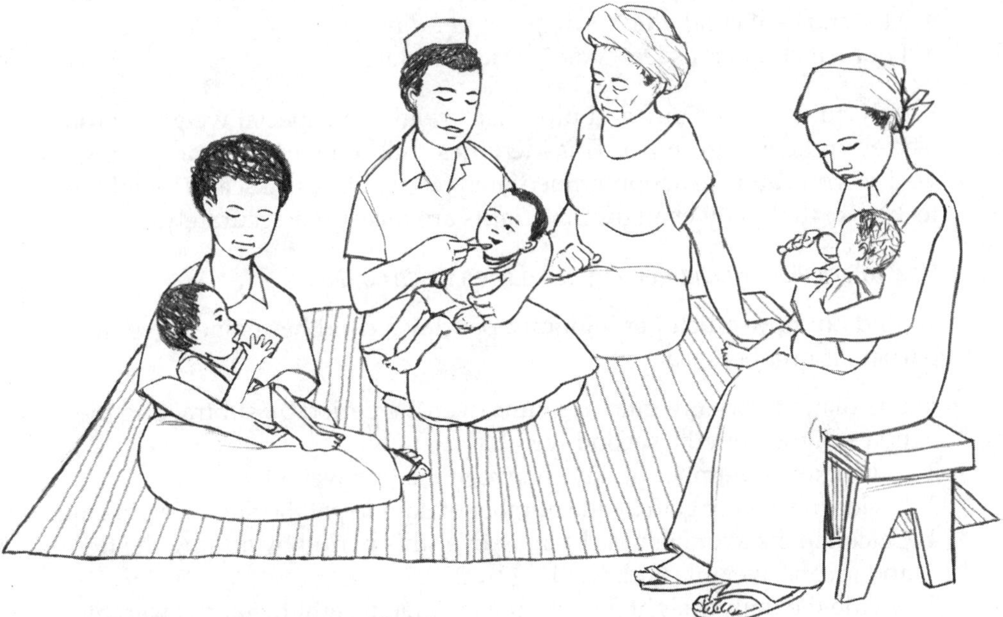

Figure 20 Feeding catch-up diets.

Show carers how to prepare enriched porridges and catch-up meals made from family foods so they can make them when they go home (see pages 66–67).

An example of a diet plan is:

6 a.m.	Catch-up formula
9 a.m.	Enriched porridge
10.30 a.m.	High energy snack
12 noon	Enriched family-food meal
3 p.m.	Catch-up formula
6 p.m.	Enriched porridge
9 p.m.	Catch-up formula
12 night	Catch-up formula

Page 50 gives more details on feeding young children and page 59 explains how to advise mothers and other carers.

Check weight gain

It takes about 4 weeks of good weight gain to rebuild the body. The best way to assess progress in the rehabilitation phase is to monitor children's daily rate of weight gain on the catch-up diet. Weight gain is:

- Good – if child gains more than 10 g/kg per day (for example a child of 5 kg gains more than 50 g/day)
- Moderate – if child gains 5–10 g/kg per day
- Poor – if child gains less than 5 g/kg per day.

Weigh children each day and plot their weights on special weight charts (see example in Figure 21). This identifies children who are not gaining well so you can take action immediately. If possible, use scales weighing to 10 g so that daily changes in weights are measured accurately.

How to calculate weight gain/kg per day on catch-up diets

To find out how much per kilogram per day a child has gained over a particular number of days:

1 Calculate the weight gain in grams over the period by subtracting the first weight from the second weight.
2 Calculate the number of days between the two weights.
3 Divide the weight gain by the number of days to get the daily weight gain.
4 Calculate the average weight in kg over this period by adding the first and second weights and dividing by 2.
5 Divide the daily weight gain by the average weight to get the weight gain/kg per day.

Example

1 Abu started catch-up formula on day 6 when he weighed 4.7 kg (4700 g). On day 16 he weighed 5.3 kg (5300 g). So he gained 5300g - 4700g = 600 g
2 The period between the two weights was day 6 to day 16 = 10 days
3 So he gained 600 g over 10 days = 60 g/day
4 His average weight in kg over this period was (4.7 + 5.3)/2 =10.0/2 = 5.0 kg
5 So Abu's weight gain/kg per day = (60 divided by 5) g/kg per day = **12 g/kg per day**. This is a good rate of weight gain.

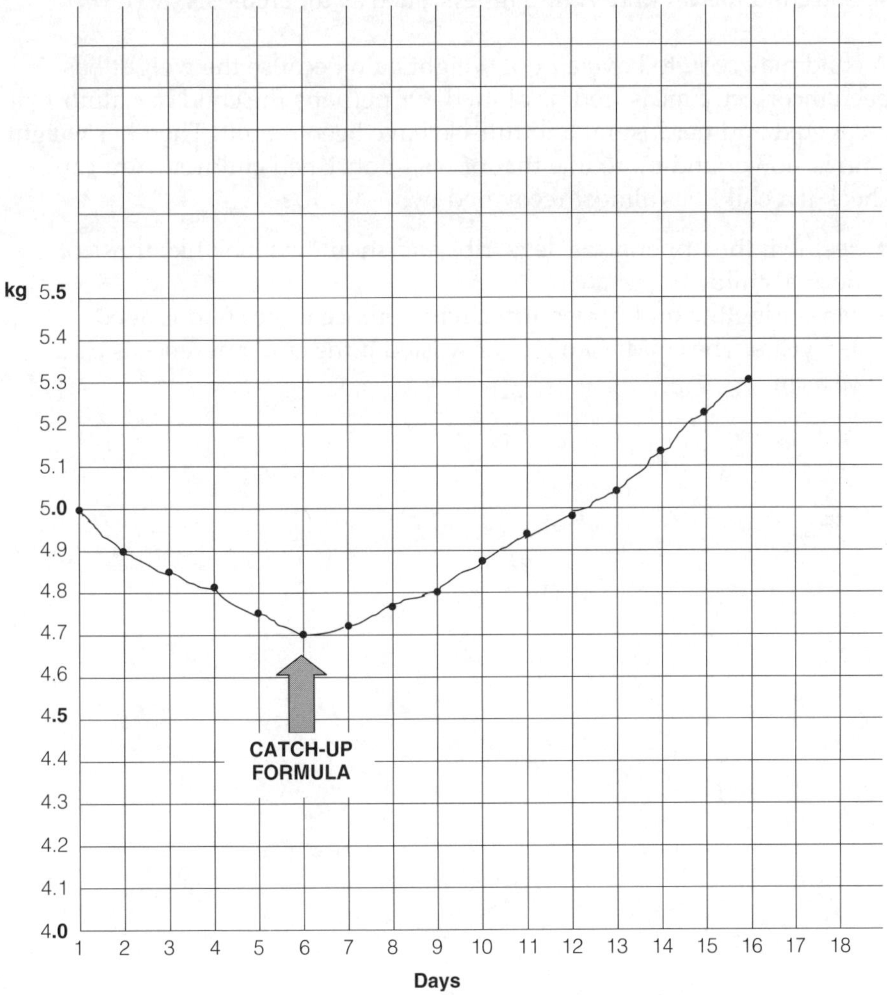

Figure 21 Abu's daily weight chart. *Make a chart like this for each child. Make the lowest weight on the vertical scale approximately 1 kg below the admission weight to allow for loss of oedema.*

Reasons for poor weight gain

Weight gain may be poor because:

- Catch-up formula is not prepared correctly
- Porridges and family meals are not enriched adequately
- The child has a poor appetite and does not eat enough (perhaps because of a new infection or unhappiness)
- The child is not fed as much as he can eat
- Carer is eating the child's food
- Feed spills onto clothes and is not replaced
- Potassium and micronutrient supplements are not given
- The child has an underlying illness, such as tuberculosis or HIV.

A child may *seem* to have a poor weight gain because the weight has been incorrectly measured or plotted. Or perhaps the child has almost recovered and her lost fat and muscle have been rebuilt. Then her weight gain is slower and more like that of well-nourished children. You can check if a child has almost recovered by:

- Seeing if the upper arms, legs, ribs and shoulders look like those of a normal child
- Measuring the mid upper arm circumference if the child is aged 1–5 years. The child is no longer wasted if the circumference is over 13.5 cm.

11 Provide loving care, play and stimulation (Step 9)

Show carers how to give loving care, play and stimulation to improve mental development.

Why malnourished children need love and stimulation

All children need extra loving care in hospital because:

- They feel frightened because everything is new and strange. They are even more frightened if their mothers or chief carers do not stay with them
- They feel ill and miserable
- They may need injections or nasogastric feeding – or they see other children having these procedures
- They hear other children crying
- They miss being picked up and cuddled; they miss their families and playmates.

Malnourished children need extra stimulation

Children learn as they explore and as people chat and play with them. When children start to move about they enjoy discovering the world around them. Severely malnourished children fall behind in their development because:

- They are weak and do not crawl or run around getting new experiences
- They are sick and are not interested in what is going on around them
- They are quiet so carers usually talk and play less with them
- Lack of nutrients may prevent their brains from developing normally
- They are usually from poor homes with few toys and little stimulation.

Delayed mental development can be the most serious long-term result of severe malnutrition. Help carers understand that playing and chatting helps children to catch up mentally and gives them a brighter future.

How to provide love and stimulation

Loving care

Children are comforted in hospital if:

- Familiar people (such as the mother) stay with them, and feed, bathe and watch over them. This also helps carers feel more useful and happy. Carers may worry that if they pick up very sick children they

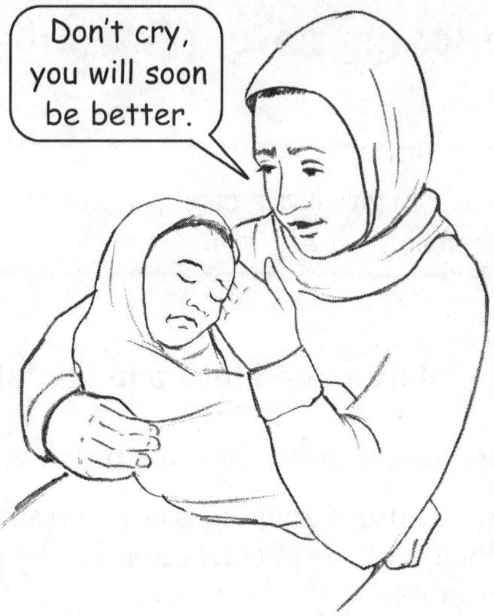

Figure 22 A sick child needs extra loving care.

might hurt them or make nurses angry. Reassure carers that holding and cuddling comforts children and has your approval
- Carers and staff look fondly at children and stroke, cuddle and talk and sing to them softly, and say their names
- They have a familiar toy or object to hold.

Do painful procedures out of sight and hearing of other children but with the carer present if possible.

Stimulation and play

Severely malnourished children may be too sick to play when first admitted but they can see and hear. Encourage carers to sing and talk lovingly to them. Make the ward as cheerful as possible by hanging colourful mobiles and pictures where children can see them. When they feel better show carers how to play little games (such as 'peep-bo' with a cloth) to stimulate them.

As children improve, give them safe objects (e.g. cups and spoons) and simple toys to play with. Tell carers to talk and play with them as much as possible. Arrange daily periods of organised play with a 'play leader' (if possible someone trained in child development or an experienced mother). The play leader should show carers individually and together how to:

- Chat and play in ways that improve children's development (see Box 11.1)
- Use everyday activities to stimulate speech and other skills. For example, when washing a child, teach words like 'water' and 'splash', blow bubbles and have fun. Teach parts of the body or names of clothes when dressing children
- Make toys that they can make at home.

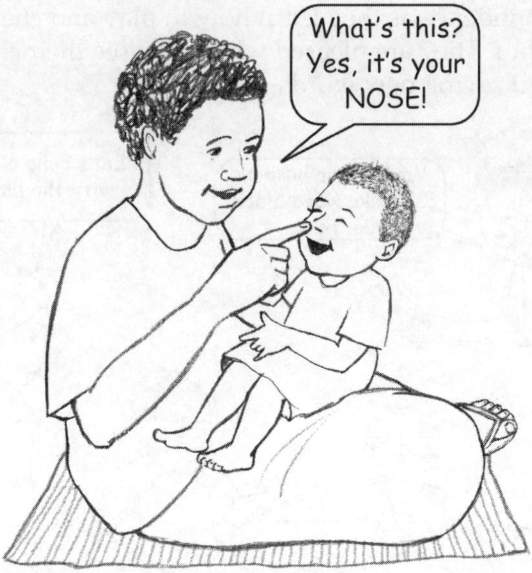

Figure 23 Teach new words.

Box 11.1 ***Organised play***

See *Management of severe malnutrition* (Appendix E page 77) for more activities.

Each play session should include movement and language activities. Activities should be appropriate for a child's stage of development. Malnourished children's mental and motor development often 'goes backward' so they may not be able to do the things that are normal for their age.

Examples of activities to improve motor development

- Help to sit by propping up with cushions
- Roll toys out of reach to encourage children to crawl to them
- Show children how to shake rattles, bang with spoons, put things in and out of containers, build with blocks and kick a ball
- Encourage children to stand by giving them something to hold on to (e.g. a chair). Encourage them to walk by holding their hands. Give them something to push along, or pull along.

Examples of activities to improve language

- Sing songs with actions (e.g. clapping hands). Play games such as counting toes
- Teach words related to activities (e.g. 'bang' when beating a can or 'bye bye' when waving goodbye)
- Play imaginary games (e.g. cuddling, feeding and talking to a doll)
- Look at and talk about pictures (e.g. make animal noises when looking at pictures of animals).

Figure 25 shows how to make simple toys. These are usually better than bought toys, which often break and are not available in many homes.

Carers gain confidence as they learn how to play and chat with children, and find it is fun. They are pleased when they see their children doing new things and saying new words.

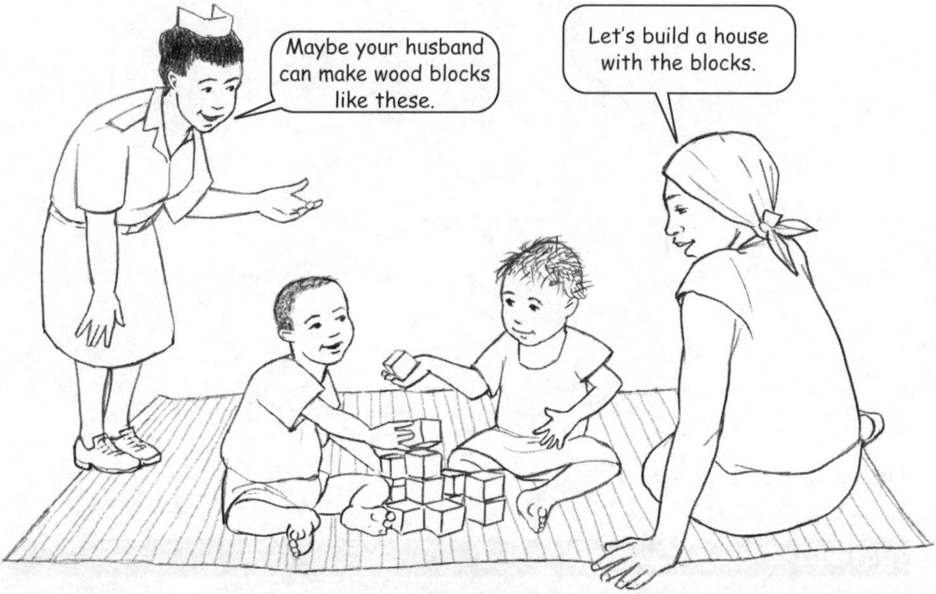

Figure 24 Play is as important as food and medicine.

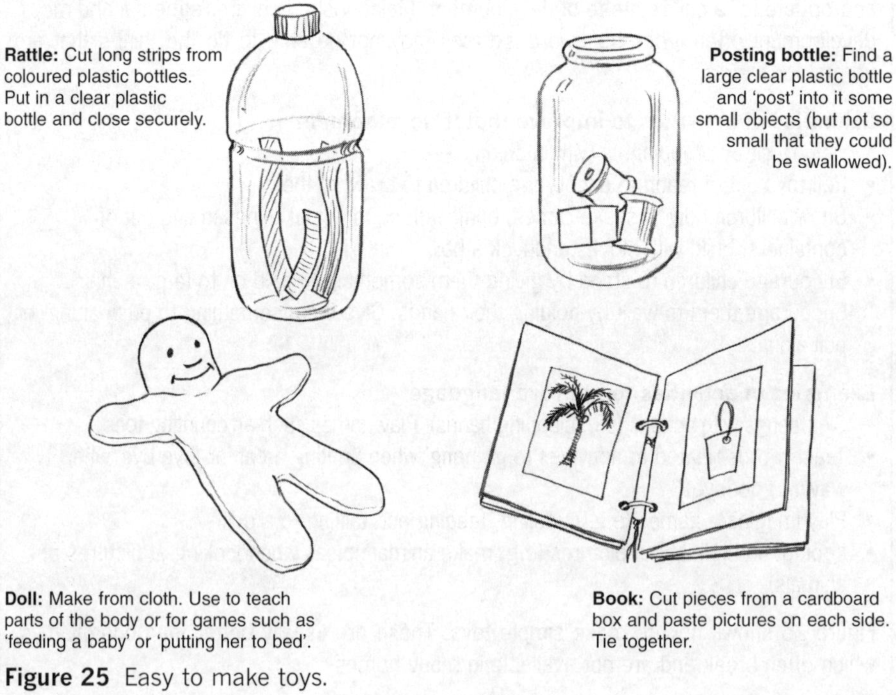

Figure 25 Easy to make toys.

12 Prepare for discharge and follow-up (Step 10)

Teach carers how to feed and care for children when they go home. Malnourished children need regular follow-up to make sure they recover fully

Deciding when a child is ready to go home

It takes about 4 weeks for a severely malnourished child to regain lost weight. It takes much longer for the immune system to be repaired. So children remain at risk of infection, relapse and death when they go home. Therefore make arrangements for adequate follow-up before children are discharged. This is even more important if children leave hospital before they have fully regained lost weight.

Children can be allowed to go home early if they:

- Have completed the transition to catch-up diets and are eating well
- Have no oedema
- Have completed antibiotic treatment
- Have received extra electrolytes and micronutrients for at least 2 weeks (or can continue at home)
- Have been gaining weight well for at least 1 week
- Can be fed catch-up diets at home
- Are up to date with their immunisations
- Have a growth chart (road-to-health-card) that has been updated
- Can be seen by a trained health worker at least weekly.

It usually takes at least 12 days for children to meet these requirements. Sometimes children may leave hospital as soon as they have completed the transition to catch-up diets if they can be referred to a 'nutrition rehabilitation unit'. Some of these units have gardens and simple kitchens so carers can learn how to produce and cook the foods their children need. To be effective, these units must have trained staff and be able to provide:

- Medical cover
- At least five catch-up meals a day
- Micronutrient supplements, mental stimulation and weight monitoring for children and education for carers.

Preparing carers and families for discharge

Try to talk with other family members before children are discharged so that they can support the mothers or carers when they go home. Make sure carers:

- Know how to feed, care for and play with their children
- Know the danger signs that indicate when to take children to a clinic urgently (see page 51)
- Know where to take the child to get immunisations, and vitamin A and other micronutrient supplements
- Have a referral letter and know where to take it.

While children are in hospital, find out their medical and family histories so that you discover why they became malnourished (see page 7). Then help the family find solutions to any problems before they are discharged. This may prevent the discharged child, and other children in the family, becoming malnourished in future.

Advise how to feed the child at home

Find out which foods the family normally eats, which ones the child likes, and other foods the family could obtain. Discuss together which mixtures of foods are best for the child. Most meals should provide:

- Extra energy. Advise adding oil, margarine, peanut butter, coconut cream or oilseeds (flours and pastes) to the staple food (e.g. thick cereal porridge, rice)
- Enough protein. Advise adding protein-rich foods that the family can afford (e.g. milk, eggs, meat, fish, fish powder, liver or other offal, groundnut paste/peanut butter, beans and/or peas)
- Enough micronutrients particularly vitamin A (e.g. from liver, red palm oil, orange-coloured fruits and vegetables), iron (e.g. from liver, red meat) and vitamin C to help the absorption of iron (e.g. from fresh fruits). Arrange for the child to get micronutrient supplements if a family cannot provide these foods. All children should receive a high dose of vitamin A every 4–6 months.

Discuss which home foods could make good snacks (e.g. bread and peanut butter, fruits, fried bean cakes). Also:

- Tell carers that the children will need frequent feeding. For example, three meals and two snacks each day plus breastfeeds (if still breastfeeding). They should give as much food as the child can eat with encouragement. Appetite is a good guide to the amounts needed if a child is well
- Show carers how to actively encourage children to eat (see Box 12.1 below)
- Make sure carers know how to practise good food and personal hygiene.

Box 12.1 *How to encourage children to eat*

Children eat more if carers supervise their meals and actively encourage them to eat in a loving way. Suggest that mothers and other family members:

- Sit and talk with children at mealtimes. Tell them the food is good; praise them as they eat
- Play games to persuade reluctant children to eat. For example, pretend to feed a doll or pet. Make mealtimes happy times
- Do not hurry children. They may eat a bit, play a bit, and then eat again
- Give children their own plates so they get their share at mealtimes
- Cut food into pieces that children can hold, and provide spoons for soft foods
- Make sure children are not thirsty. Thirsty children eat less. But do not fill up their stomachs with too much drink before or during the meal
- Never force feed. This increases stress and decreases appetite. If children refuse food, take it away and offer it later
- Give special love and attention if children are unhappy (e.g. is grieving for a lost relative).

Box 12.2 page 54 describes the special feeding and care HIV+ children need. The publications *Complementary feeding: family foods for breastfed children* and *HIV/AIDS: a guide for nutrition, care and support* listed in Appendix E page 78 give more information on feeding young children including those with HIV/AIDS.

Show how to stimulate and play with a child at home

Make sure carers know how to stimulate children's development by talking and playing with them, including during everyday activities (see pages 46–48). Discuss together which play activities are best for their children. Help carers think how to put these ideas into practice, and which objects can be used as toys. Show them how to make simple safe toys (see Figure 25 page 48).

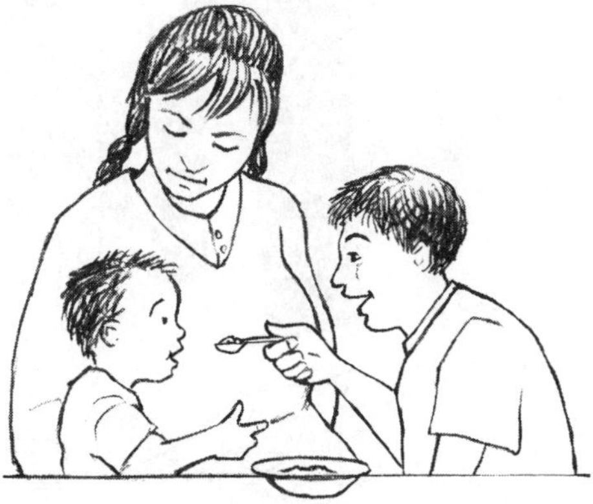

Figure 26 Encourage a child to eat.

Teach the danger signs of infection and relapse

Tell carers to take children quickly to the clinic if they develop any of the following signs:

- Not eating
- Fever

- Convulsions
- Cough with fast breathing or chest indrawing
- Very frequent watery stools or stools with blood
- Diarrhoea for more than 14 days
- Oedema.

Explain that children need regular follow-up

Tell carers to take children to their local clinic for weighing and follow-up when they go home.

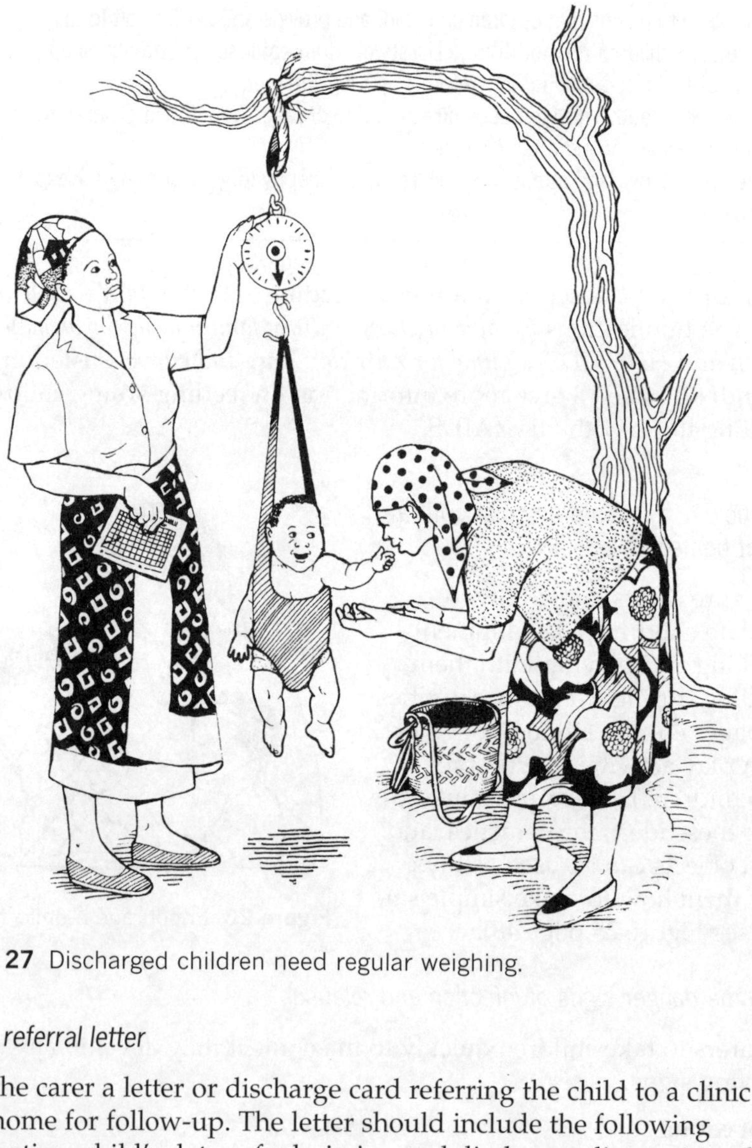

Figure 27 Discharged children need regular weighing.

Give a referral letter

Give the carer a letter or discharge card referring the child to a clinic near their home for follow-up. The letter should include the following information: child's dates of admission and discharge; diagnosis and inpatient treatment; weight on discharge; present diet; advice given on feeding and play; reasons for the child becoming malnourished; recommendations for continuing care (e.g. diet, play, medicines, micronutrients, frequency of follow-up needed).

Caring for children after discharge

There should be follow-up programmes for discharged children so that they:

- Are visited at home by community health workers *and/or*
- Visit their nearest young child clinic or return to the hospital for frequent weighing and follow-up.

Keep in *regular* contact with the clinic to check if discharged children are being followed up and growing well. Then hospital staff can assess their treatment and advice, and take action if needed.

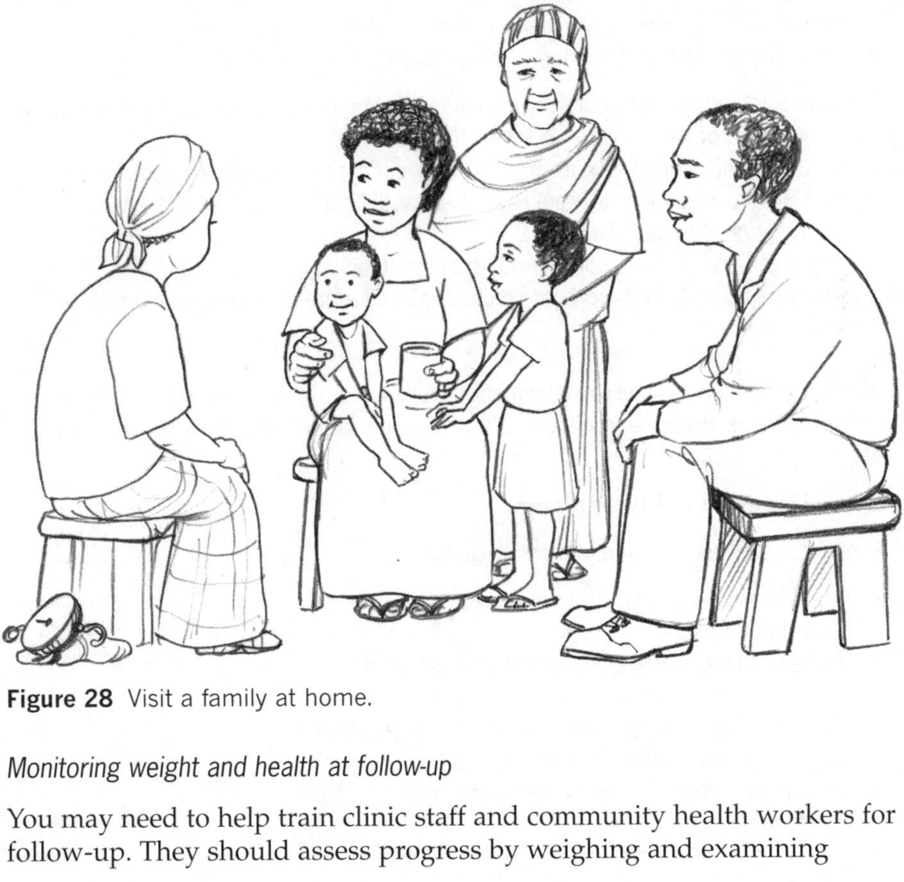

Figure 28 Visit a family at home.

Monitoring weight and health at follow-up

You may need to help train clinic staff and community health workers for follow-up. They should assess progress by weighing and examining children weekly for at least the first month and then regularly according to the local schedule. They should praise the carer if the child is gaining weight well. If a child has poor weight gain, a health worker should:

1 Ask what the child is eating, how often and if someone is encouraging the child to eat.
2 Ask about the child's health and examine her. Look for infection.
3 Ask the carer why she thinks the child has not gained weight.
4 Send the child for further examination if necessary.

When the reason for poor progress is known, the health worker should:

1 Treat any infections; give deworming medicine if necessary.
2 Discuss with the family how they can feed and care for the child better.
3 Help families overcome any food shortages (e.g. enrol the child in a feeding programme) or other problems affecting family nutrition.

Box 12.2 ***Feeding and caring for HIV+ children***

Children who are HIV+ may become malnourished and ill again because:

- The HIV virus damages the immune system
- The mother or other relatives may be HIV+ and so less able to care for the child.

Good feeding can prevent poor growth in the early stages of the infection and may delay the progression of HIV to AIDS. So HIV+ children should:

- Receive as much good food as possible and be fed more frequently than usual. Ill children may need foods that are easy to eat and digest (see below) and extra encouragement to eat (see Box 12.1)
- Be weighed regularly so poor growth is identified quickly
- Be treated quickly for infections. Common infections are diarrhoea, sore mouth and pneumonia.

All HIV+ children need multi-micronutrient supplements. Do not give iron as this makes some infections worse. Advise the family to be especially careful about hygiene as HIV+ children get infections easily.

Special foods for ill HIV+ children

Foods that are easy to eat and digest include:

- Fermented and soured milks (e.g. yogurt)
- Fermented porridge
- Mashed banana, avocado, mango and pawpaw
- Skinned, mashed, well-cooked pulses (e.g. lentils)
- Mashed pumpkin, and potatoes and other root vegetables
- Minced or mashed meat and chicken, and pounded fish
- Smooth groundnut or other oilseed paste, peanut butter
- Cold foods.

▶

Box 12.2 ***Continued***

Foods that *sometimes* cause digestive problems include:

- Wholemeal (brown) cereals
- Very fatty foods or fried foods
- Hot, spicy or very sweet foods.

13 Support mothers and other carers

Mothers and other carers are essential members of the team caring for severely malnourished children. They can do a lot to help their children recover in the ward and at home. So it is important that all carers know what they are meant to do and that they feel comfortable and able to talk with ward staff.

Carers learn best if:

1 You are friendly, polite, and listen sympathetically to their fears, opinions and problems.
2 You adjust your teaching and counselling to their levels of knowledge. Always check that your advice is feasible and has been understood.
3 You do not give too much information at one time, especially when a mother has just arrived and is anxious. Tell her only what she needs to know at the time. During the stabilisation phase, gently and privately ask about her family situation and give relevant advice as you attend her child. When children start to improve most carers enjoy learning together.
4 All staff give consistent advice. So prepare this advice with colleagues, including those working in the community, and make sure all staff know and understand it. Remember carers get information from junior staff and other carers in the ward. Carers watch what you are doing, so check that ward procedures are good examples of how to feed, care for, and play with young children.
5 You demonstrate how to feed and care for children. For example, show how to prepare meals, how to practise good hygiene and how to talk with children. After demonstrating an activity ask one or more carers to repeat it.

During the stabilisation phase

We explain how to care for the carer on admission on page 9. When the carer has settled in, tell her what is wrong with her child (see below) and the treatment he will get. Be careful not to blame the carer for the child's illness.

Explain the child's illness

Explain that the child is sick because he has not been eating enough. He may have an infection. This is why he looks thin (and swollen – if there is oedema), has a poor appetite and is unhappy and not playful. Tell her this illness is called 'severe malnutrition' (use the local word if there is one). Reassure her that we expect the child to start to improve in a few days.

Explain about keeping the child warm

Explain the child easily becomes cold because he has lost a lot of fat. Fat is like a blanket that keeps us warm. If a child has swelling (oedema), explain that this is fluid (not fat) and so does not keep the child warm.

Tell the carer she can help by:

- Dressing the child in warm clothes
- Keeping him covered with a blanket
- Keeping him dry by changing nappies and bedding as soon as they are wet
- Sleeping with him.

Explain about feeding

Explain that the child's body is weak and not working properly. This means the child:

- Cannot digest ordinary food or large amounts at one time. So the child needs to be fed *small* amounts but *very often* and must be fed *day and night*. Explain that children often die at night if they are not fed regularly. Tell the carer that her child will get a special milk drink and extra vitamins. Reassure her that the amount of milk you give will be enough. Too much at this stage would be harmful. If the child is too sick to drink, staff will give the milk through a tube passed through his nose
- Needs a sugary milk drink to help his brain work properly. If the child becomes drowsy (abnormally sleepy) this is a sign that the brain lacks food
- Has too much salt in his body so should not have salty food.

Tell the carer she can help by:

- Feeding her child every 2–3 hours day and night. Tell her to start feeding as soon as the nurse gives her the milk. Ask her to make sure the child drinks all the milk and none is spilt. Show her how to put a saucer under the child's chin to catch any dribbled milk and refeed it (see Figure 16 page 36). Tell her not to give the milk too fast or the child may vomit. If the child does vomit she should tell the nurse. She should keep any leftovers as the nurse records what the child drinks
- Breastfeeding whenever the child wants – after giving the special milk. The child must get all the special milk first

- Not sharing her own food with the child. It may be too strong or too salty and make the child worse.

Warn that feeding may take a long time but it is one of the most important things carers can do, especially in the first few days and at night.

Explain the need for loving care

Explain that, as well as feeling ill and miserable, the child is probably frightened because everything is new and strange. Tell the carer she can comfort the child by gently cuddling and stroking him, by softly talking and singing to him and by saying his name. Explain that she can help other children and carers in the ward by smiling and talking with them.

Explain when to call a nurse quickly

Explain that a child's condition can get worse very suddenly. If this happens the child needs urgent attention. Tell the carer she can help by watching her child carefully. She must immediately call a member of staff if he feels cold or becomes limp or drowsy and hard to wake up.

Explain how to prevent infections

Explain to the carer that the child will be given antibiotics to cure infections. To prevent new infections, staff are careful to keep themselves and the ward as clean as possible.

Tell the carer she can help to prevent infections spreading by:

- Washing her hands thoroughly with soap: *after* using the toilet or touching soiled nappies, clothes or bed linen; *before* preparing food or feeding her child and *before and after* touching another child in the ward
- Keeping her child clean, changing nappies when soiled and putting them in the correct place
- Keeping food and utensils covered, and washing utensils with soap
- Not feeding other children with the same spoon that she used to feed her child.

Explain about watery diarrhoea

If the child has diarrhoea, explain that he may become dehydrated (too dry). That is why you are giving him extra drinks. The child should sip this special drink slowly but he must drink it all even if it takes a long time. Staff will give the drink through a tube passed through the nose if the child becomes too sick to drink.

Tell the carer she can help by making sure the child drinks all the special drink.

During the rehabilitation phase

Point out that the child is starting to eat well and to smile. These are signs of recovery. The carer will feel happier as she sees these signs. Congratulate her on her care of the child.

Explain about feeding stronger food so the child gains weight quickly

Explain that the child can now have a 'stronger' milk drink and eat other food, although it must not be salty. This will make him gain weight quickly.

Tell the carer she can help by encouraging the child to eat as much as possible (after the first 2 days on the stronger diet) and to ask for more if needed. Remind her not to share her own food with the child. It may be too salty.

Explain about playing with the child

The carer will have noticed that the child is more alert. Tell her that now he needs extra attention and stimulation. This will help make him a happier and cleverer child. All children learn faster if people talk and play with them. Explain that play is as important as good food and medicine.

Show the carer how to play with her child in ways that encourage him to talk, to learn new skills and to move more (and so strengthen his weak body). Involve her in play activities so that she gains confidence.

Encourage the carer to continue to talk and play with the child like this when she goes home as it takes a long time for the child's mental ability to recover. Discuss how other family members might help. Show her how to make simple toys that encourage mental and physical development.

Example of a wall chart made by nurses
(to remind staff how to care for severely malnourished children)

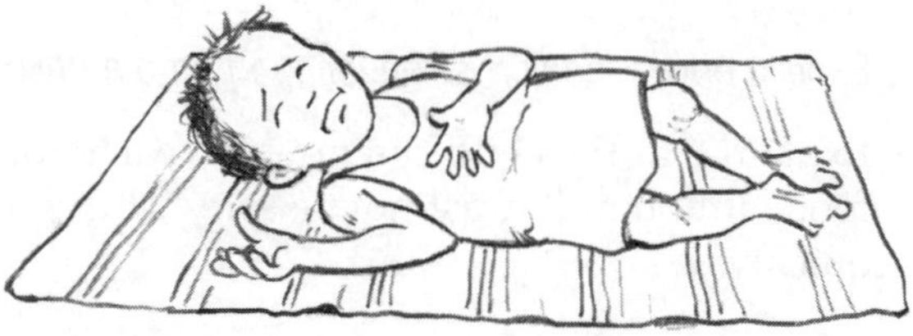

I am very malnourished so:

- I do not want to eat
- My blood sugar falls quickly if I do not eat often
- I get cold easily
- My gut, kidneys, liver, heart and cells do not work properly
- My body contains too much salt and too little potassium
- My infections are hidden
- I feel ill, weak, frightened and miserable.

To make me better, please:

- Keep me warm
- Give me the special starter milk drink
- Feed me every 3 hours day and night
- Give me antibiotics and extra potassium
- Give me extra vitamin A and other micronutrients (but not iron yet)
- Do not give me too much fluid
- Give me lots of love and attention.

Now I am starting to feel better. See, I am smiling and playing.
And I am very hungry. So please:

- Give me catch-up formula so I gain weight fast
- Feed me often and at night
- Give me as much as I can eat
- Keep giving me extra micronutrients including iron, and potassium
- Play with me so I can learn faster
- Tell my family how to care for me when we go home.

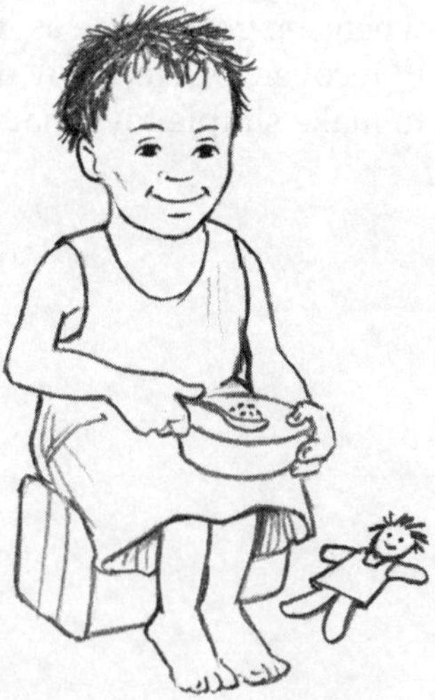

Appendix

A Equipment and supplies

The following lists the *ideal* ward, kitchen and pharmacy equipment and supplies needed. Starred* items are *essential* for successfully treating severe malnutrition.

For the ward

Malnutrition treatment guidelines*
Glucostix/Dextrostix and glucometer
Thermometer (preferably low-reading)*
Child weighing scales (preferably reading to 10 g)*
Pan-type scale/sling to weigh very ill children
Graph or squared paper for weight charts*
Fluid intake/output charts*
Temperature/pulse/respiration charts*
Paediatric nasogastric tubes*
Syringes/needles/cannulas*
Paediatric giving set*
Glucose/dextrose or sugar*
Oxygen*
Oxygen mask/nasal prongs*
Hot water
Soap/chlorhexidine spray*
Paper towels
Heater
Nappies, bed linen, blankets*
Toys* (preferably low cost that can be made at home)
Food and utensils, washing facilities, mattresses, etc. for carers*
Unbroken windows

For the kitchen

Recipes (preferably laminated as a wall chart) for starter and catch-up formula using the type of milk available and for different volumes (e.g. for $1\frac{1}{2}$, 2, $2\frac{1}{2}$ and 3 litres)*
Refrigerator

Stove
Electric food blender or whisk*
Containers/jugs with ½ and 1 litre mark for making up feeds*
Container to measure liquid milk if used (reading to 10 ml)*
Medicine cup with 5 ml divisions*
Dietary scale (easy-to-read to 5 g) or calibrated measuring containers (see Appendix B pages 67 and 68)*
Feeding cups and spoons*
5 ml spoon
Milk: powder, fresh or longlife*
Vegetable oil*
Sugar*
Ingredients for modified family meals for catch-up diets (see pages 41 and 50, and Appendix B pages 66–67)*

For the pharmacy

Oral rehydration salts (ORS) or **Re**hydration **so**lution for **mal**nutrition (ReSoMal) packets*
Multivitamin mix*
Electrolyte/mineral or potassium chloride (KCl) solution or Slow K*
Iron*
Folic acid*
High dose vitamin A*
Metronidazole*
Co-trimoxazole*
Ampicillin*
Amoxicillin*
Gentamicin*
Chloramphenicol*
Mebendazole*
Measles vaccine*
Tine/Mantoux test
Zinc and castor oil ointment or tulle gras
Potassium permanganate crystals
½ strength Darrow's with 5% dextrose or Ringer's lactate with 5% dextrose, or half-normal saline with 5% dextrose, or Ringer's lactate*
50% glucose or 10% glucose (sterile ampoules for IV)*
Ampoules of sterile water*
Furosemide*

Appendix

B Recipes

Electrolyte/mineral solution

Ingredient	*Amount (g)*
Potassium chloride	224
Tripotassium citrate	81
Magnesium chloride	76
Zinc acetate	8.2
Copper sulphate	1.4
Water	To 2500 ml

Preparation

- Dissolve ingredients in cooled boiled water
- Store in sterilised bottles in a refrigerator if possible
- Discard if solution turns cloudy
- Make fresh at least each month.

If it is not possible to make this solution give potassium, magnesium and zinc separately (see pages 24 and 32).

Premixed packets of these electrolytes and minerals are available commercially from Nutriset (see address page 77). Nutriset packets also contain folic acid and multivitamins so there is no need to give these as separate additions as indicated on page 32. Do give the large dose of vitamin A on Day 1 (and on Days 2 and 14 if there is xerophthalmia) and iron in the rehabilitation phase.

Starter formulas

The following recipes make 1000 ml (one litre) of starter formula. They contain 75 kcal and 0.9 g protein per 100 ml.

How to prepare

Weigh or measure the ingredients, including the water, as accurately as possible; otherwise the feed may be too dilute or too strong. We describe below how to use volume measures if you do not have dietary scales. Remember that germs grow quickly in milk feeds so wash your hands thoroughly with soap before preparing feeds. Make sure that utensils and kitchen surfaces are very clean.

Starter formula: using full cream fresh or long-life milk

Full cream fresh or long-life milk	300 ml
Sugar	100 g
Oil	20 g
Electrolyte/mineral solution	20 ml
Water	To 1000 ml

Starter formula: using full cream milk powder

Full cream milk powder	35 g
Sugar	100 g
Oil	20 g
Electrolyte/mineral solution	20 ml
Water (880 ml)	To 1000 ml

Starter formula: using skimmed milk powder

Skimmed milk powder	25 g
Sugar	100 g
Oil	30 g
Electrolyte/mineral solution	20 ml
Water (880 ml)	To 1000 ml

Using an electric blender:

1 Before starting, boil and cool water and fresh milk (if used).
2 If using milk powder, put enough water in the blender to cover the blades (to stop the powder sticking to them).
3 Measure or weigh the milk and put in blender.
4 Measure or weigh the sugar and put in blender.
5 Measure or weigh the oil and put in blender. Oil sticks to surfaces of containers, so use a small container for measuring/weighing and rinse out with a little water. Add this to blender.
6 Add 20 ml electrolyte/mineral solution .
7 Add water *up to* the one litre mark.

8 Blend the ingredients. Do this in short bursts to prevent the milk frothing out and spilling.

Using a whisk (or fork):

1 Before starting, boil and cool water and fresh milk (if used).
2 Weigh or measure the sugar and oil. Mix together thoroughly (this helps to prevent the oil separating out).
3 Weigh or measure the milk and add. Mix well.
4 Add 20 ml electrolyte/mineral solution. Mix well.
5 Add water *up to* the one litre mark, and whisk vigorously.
6 Whisk vigorously before feeding if oil has separated out.

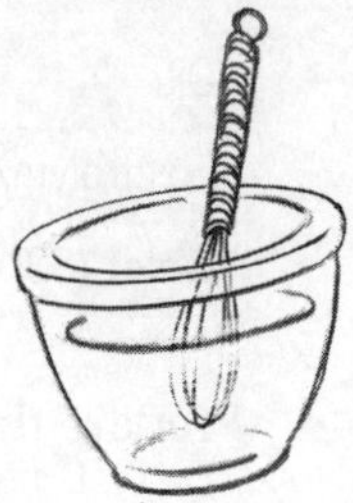

Figure 29
Whisk well to prevent oil separating out.

Keep the feed covered and in a refrigerator if possible. Throw away any feed not used after 12 hours. If there is no refrigerator make smaller quantities (e.g. 500 ml or enough for two feeds). Do not keep longer than 2 hours.

Catch-up formulas

The following recipes make 1000 ml (one litre) of catch-up formula. Each recipe contains 100 kcal and 3 g protein per 100 ml.

Catch-up formula: using full cream fresh or long-life milk

Full cream fresh or long-life milk	880 ml
Sugar	75 g
Oil	20 g
Electrolyte/mineral solution	20 ml
Water	To 1000 ml

Catch-up formula: using full cream milk powder

Full cream milk powder	110 g
Sugar	50 g
Oil	30 g
Electrolyte/mineral solution	20 ml
Water (830 ml)	To 1000 ml

Catch-up formula: using skimmed milk powder

Skimmed milk powder	80 g
Sugar	50 g
Oil	60 g
Electrolyte/mineral solution	20 ml
Water (830 ml)	To 1000 ml

Prepare these in the same way as starter formula.

Catch-up diets

Recipes for catch-up diets using local foods (also see page 50)

The following recipes provide enough energy (200 kcal) and protein (6 g) for one meal for a child weighing up to 10 kg. This assumes that the child has 7 feeds or meals each 24 hours.

Catch-up meal: porridge with groundnuts

	Amounts	
Ingredients	*For one child*	*For 5 children*
Cereal flour	20 g	100 g
Groundnut/oilseed paste	20 g	100 g
Sugar	10 g	50 g
Make a *thick* porridge with the cereal flour and then stir in the groundnut paste and sugar.		

Catch-up meal: porridge with milk (cow/goat/sheep)

	Amounts	
Ingredients	*For one child*	*For 5 children*
Cereal flour	25 g	125 g
Milk	120 ml	600 ml
Sugar	15 g	75 g
Oil/margarine	5 g	25 g
Make a *thick* porridge, replacing most of the water with milk. (Or use 15 g whole milk powder instead of 120 ml fresh milk). Then add the oil and sugar.		

Catch-up meal of rice, legumes, pumpkin, egg and margarine

	For one child		For 5 children	
Ingredients	*Weight (g)*	*Volume*	*Weight (g)*	*Volume*
Rice (cooked)	90	4½ big spoons	450	22½ big spoons
Beans/peas/dhall (cooked, mashed)	30	1½ big spoons	150	7½ big spoons
Pumpkin (cooked, mashed)	30	1½ big spoons	150	7½ big spoons
Egg	30	1 egg	150	5 eggs
Margarine	10	2 teaspoons	50	10 teaspoons
Big spoon = rounded 10 ml spoon. Teaspoon = 5 ml spoon. Prepare meal in the local way. Do not make too watery.				

These recipes can be used for home catch-up meals. Increase the amounts if the child can eat more. There are more recipes for feeding young children at home in *Complementary feeding: family foods for breastfed children* (see Appendix E page 78) and *The management of severe malnutrition in Uganda*, 1999, Ministry of Health, Uganda. Carers should know that meals must not be watery. They must contain enough energy and nutrients in volumes that small children can eat.

Ready-to-use formulas and food-aid ingredients

A starter formula called F-75 and a catch-up formula called F-100 may be available from UNICEF (ask your UNICEF Country Office). They are available commercially from Nutriset (see address on page 77) who are also developing catch-up diets that may be suitable for home use.

Some 'food-aid' foods (some fortified with micronutrients) can be used as ingredients for ward and home catch-up diets. For details see *HIV/AIDS: a guide to nutrition, care and support* (page 78).

How to change weights of foods to volumes

Method A

1 Choose the minimum number of litres of each formula you will need to prepare at one time. Below we use 2 litres of starter formula as an example.
2 Weigh the sugar needed for the recipe (e.g. 200 g if making 2 litres of starter formula). Use dietary or pharmacy scales (accurate to 1 g).

3 Find a container that holds exactly this amount when filled to the brim. *Or,* if you cannot find a container that holds the exact amount, try to find one that holds exactly half, or a third, or a quarter of the amount needed (e.g. 100 g, or 66 g, or 50 g sugar).
Or, find two containers that together give the amount needed (e.g. 190 g + 10 g sugar).
4 Write the ingredient and amount on the container (e.g. Sugar 200 g) with permanent ink or paint so it will not wash off.
5 Now weigh the milk powder and repeat the process.
6 Transfer the quantities to the ward recipe (see example below).

For oil, the volume in millilitres (ml) is almost the same as the weight in grams (g). A medicine cup is suitable for measuring oil or electrolyte/ mineral solution.

Example of recipe for 2 litres of starter formula using local measures:

	Required weight or volume	*Local measure*
Full cream milk powder	70 g	1 yogurt pot + 2 red scoops
Sugar	200 g	1 tin
Oil	40 g	40 ml
Electrolyte/mineral solution	40 ml	40 ml
Water (1760 ml)	To 2000 ml	To 2000 ml

Useful tips:

- Although time-consuming, organising measuring containers only needs to be done once. It is worth taking time to find containers of exactly the right volume. Then you simply fill up and level the food with the back of a knife. The needed amount is now ready to use
- Choose strong containers that will not lose shape. They hold less if dented
- Always label the container so you know for which food it is to be used, and how much it holds.

Method B

1 Choose the minimum number of litres of each formula you will need to prepare at one time. Below we use one litre of catch-up formula as an example.
2 Weigh the ingredient (e.g. 50 g sugar) needed for the recipe using scales accurate to 1 g.

3 Pour into a measuring container with 5 ml divisions (e.g. a medicine cup).
4 Read the volume.
5 Repeat several times to check if the volume is always the same. If so, write on the ward recipe.

Example:

Sugar	50 g	60 ml

6 Repeat for the other ingredients.

Useful tip: Different types of sugar have different volumes. The same is true for different types and brands of milk powder. So always do these conversions with the ingredients you will be using.

Appendix

C Feeding charts

Chart 1 Amounts of starter formula for children of different weights

Amount of starter formula needed at each 3-hourly feed (8 feeds/day) *					
For most children (i.e. no oedema, oedema + or oedema ++)			***For children with severe oedema (i.e. oedema +++)***		
Child's weight on admission (kg)	***Amount at each 3-hourly feed (ml)***	***Give NG feeds if intake over 24 hours is less than: (ml)***	*Child's oedematous weight on admission (kg)*	*Amount at each 3-hourly feed (ml)*	*Give NG feeds if intake over 24 hours is less than: (ml)*
2.0	**30**	**210**	2.0	25	160
2.2	**35**	**230**	2.2	30	180
2.4	**40**	**250**	2.4	30	190
2.6	**45**	**270**	2.6	35	210
2.8	**45**	**290**	2.8	35	220
3.0	**50**	**320**	3.0	40	240
3.2	**55**	**340**	3.2	40	250
3.4	**55**	**360**	3.4	45	270
3.6	**60**	**380**	3.6	45	290
3.8	**60**	**400**	3.8	50	300
4.0	**65**	**420**	4.0	50	320
4.2	**70**	**440**	4.2	55	340
4.4	**70**	**460**	4.4	55	350
4.6	**75**	**490**	4.6	60	370
4.8	**80**	**510**	4.8	60	380
5.0	**80**	**530**	5.0	65	400
5.2	**85**	**550**	5.2	65	420
5.4	**90**	**570**	5.4	70	430

* Use these amounts on Day 1 and then keep the volume the same until the child is ready to transfer to the catch-up formula. Amounts rounded to 5 ml.
NG = nasogastric

▶

Amount of starter formula needed at each 3-hourly feed (8 feeds/day) *					
For most children (i.e. no oedema, oedema + or oedema ++)			*For children with severe oedema (i.e. oedema +++)*		
Child's weight on admission (kg)	**Amount at each 3-hourly feed (ml)**	**Give NG feeds if intake over 24 hours is less than: (ml)**	Child's oedematous weight on admission (kg)	Amount at each 3-hourly feed (ml)	Give NG feeds if intake over 24 hours is less than:(ml)
5.6	**90**	**590**	5.6	70	450
5.8	**95**	**610**	5.8	75	460
6.0	**100**	**640**	6.0	75	480
6.2	**100**	**660**	6.2	80	500
6.4	**105**	**680**	6.4	80	510
6.6	**110**	**700**	6.6	85	530
6.8	**110**	**720**	6.8	85	540
7.0	**115**	**740**	7.0	90	560
7.2	**120**	**760**	7.2	90	570
7.4	**120**	**780**	7.4	95	590
7.6	**125**	**810**	7.6	95	610
7.8	**130**	**830**	7.8	100	620
8.0	**130**	**850**	8.0	100	640
8.2	**135**	**870**	8.2	105	650
8.4	**140**	**890**	8.4	105	670
8.6	**140**	**910**	8.6	110	690
8.8	**145**	**930**	8.8	110	700
9.0	**145**	**950**	9.0	115	720
9.2	**150**	**980**	9.2	115	730
9.4	**155**	**1000**	9.4	120	750
9.6	**155**	**1030**	9.6	120	770
9.8	**160**	**1040**	9.8	125	780
10.0	**160**	**1060**	10.0	125	780

* Use these amounts on Day 1 and then keep the volume the same until the child is ready to transfer to the catch-up formula. Amounts rounded to 5 ml.
NG = nasogastric

Chart 2 Daily ward feeding chart

Prepare this chart each day so that you know how much each child should receive at each feed and how much of each formula to prepare.

- For children on starter formula, use Chart 1 to find out the amounts needed by each child at each 3-hourly feed. Then calculate the amount each child should take over 24 hours. This tells you how much formula to prepare. To calculate the amounts needed if the child is fed 2-hourly see page 36
- For children on catch-up formula, see page 40 for the amounts needed. After the 3-day transition period allow a little extra at each feed so the child can have more if still hungry.

Example (also see pages 35 and 36):

Date: 6 August

	Starter formula prescribed				Milk-based catch-up formula prescribed		
Name	**Number feeds over 24 hours**	**Amount of each feed (ml)**	**Total over 24 hours (ml)**	**Name**	**Number feeds over 24 hours**	**Amount of each feed (ml)**	**Total over 24 hours (ml)**
Kofi	8	90	720	Meena[1]	8	65	520
Grace	8	100	800	Charles[2]	7	140+	More than 980
Thandi	12	40	480				
Kim	12	70	840				
Total			2800				1500+

1 Transition Day 1 for Meena.
2 Two days after the transition period for Charles. Yesterday he ate 130 ml at his last feed.

Chart 3 Example of a child's daily feed intake and output chart

(for 3-hourly feeds of starter formula)

Make a chart like this for each child each day; record the amounts at each feed.

Name: *Grace* Date: 6 Aug Day: 2

Weight on admission (kg): 7.8 Oedema on admission: +++

Formula: Starter Amount to feed 3-hourly (ml): 100

Time	Type of feed	Amount offered (ml)	Amount left over (ml)	Amount taken (ml)	Vomit (ml)	Watery stool (Y = yes)
9am	Starter	100	20	80	0	
12 noon	Starter	100	20	80	0	Y ReSoMal
3pm	Starter	100	50	50	0	
6pm	Starter	100	100	0	0	
9pm	Starter	100	50	50	0	Y ReSoMal
12 night	Starter	100	20	80	80	
3am	Starter	100	100	0	0	
6am	Starter	100	100	0	0	
Total		800	410	390	80	

Total taken and not vomited 390 - 80 = 310 ml

Grace has taken and not vomited 310 ml, which is less than the minimum amount needed (620 ml see Chart 1). She refused her last 2 feeds so should be fed by nasogastric tube.

Appendix

D Checklist to monitor care of severely malnourished children

Use this checklist to monitor the care given to severely malnourished children in your ward.

In outpatients

- Are all severely malnourished children brought to the front of the queue so they can be admitted quickly?
- Have the doctors, clinical officers, nurses in outpatients (as well as ward staff) been trained about treatment of severe malnutrition? Have they written guidelines?

On admission

Are all severely malnourished children:

- Examined quickly but carefully?
- Immediately given any emergency treatment needed?
- *Not* given IV fluids except in shock?
- Fed immediately?

Stabilisation phase

Are all severely malnourished children:

- Fed every 3 hours day and night (or 2-hourly if hypoglycaemic or hypothermic)?
- Given special 'starter formula' in the correct amount (based on admission weight)?
- Fed by nasogastric tube if refusing or vomiting all or most of their feed?
- If breastfeeding, breastfed between feeds of starter formula?
- Kept warm and dry all the time?
- Given extra potassium and magnesium (or electrolyte/mineral solution) daily?
- *Not* given salt?
- Given zinc and copper (or electrolyte/mineral solution) daily?

- Given a high dose of vitamin A on day 1?
- Given folic acid daily?
- Given multivitamin syrup daily?
- *Not* given iron?
- Given broad-spectrum antibiotics from Day 1?
- Given loving care?
- Weighed daily?
- Transferred to the catch-up formula as soon as appetite returns and most of the oedema has gone?

Are dehydrated children given ReSoMal and rehydrated slower than usual?

Do ward staff:

- Record amount of rehydration fluid given?
- Monitor pulse and respiration rates when giving IV fluid (every 5–10 minutes) or oral rehydration (at least every hour)?
- Give antibiotics on time?
- Use the correct recipes for the starter (and catch-up) formulas?
- Mix feeds thoroughly so the oil does not separate out?
- Make feeds *up to* the one litre mark (*not* 1 litre of water added)?
- Keep a daily intake record for each child for each feed (amount offered, left over, eaten) and an output record (vomit and watery stools)?
- Wash hands before touching a child?
- Keep the ward clean to avoid cross-infections?
- Make the ward cheerful with pictures and toys?

Are carers:

- Welcomed to the ward and given information about facilities?
- Asked privately about their family backgrounds and problems, and history of their children's illnesses?
- Told about their children's illness and shown how to feed and care for them?
- Told not to share their food with their children?
- Told about the importance of hygiene to stop cross-infection?

Rehabilitation phase

Are all children:

- Fed the correct amount of catch-up formula during the 3-day transitional phase?
- After this, actively encouraged to eat as much as possible?
- Given catch-up formula or a catch-up diet 7 times a day?
- Given iron in addition to electrolytes and other micronutrients?
- Weighed daily to monitor weight gain?

- Talked and played with by carers and staff?
- Given periods of organised play and stimulation?
- Given any needed immunisations?

Are carers:

- Shown how to talk and play with children in ways that improve development?
- Shown how to feed and care for children at home?
- Told the danger signs of infection and relapse?
- Told where and when to take their children for regular weighing and follow-up?
- Given a referral letter?

Do staff check that discharged children are attending a clinic regularly and gaining weight?

Assessing progress

- What percentage of malnourished children die during hospital treatment?
- What percentages of children gain weight at the 'good', 'moderate' and 'poor' rates during rehabilitation?

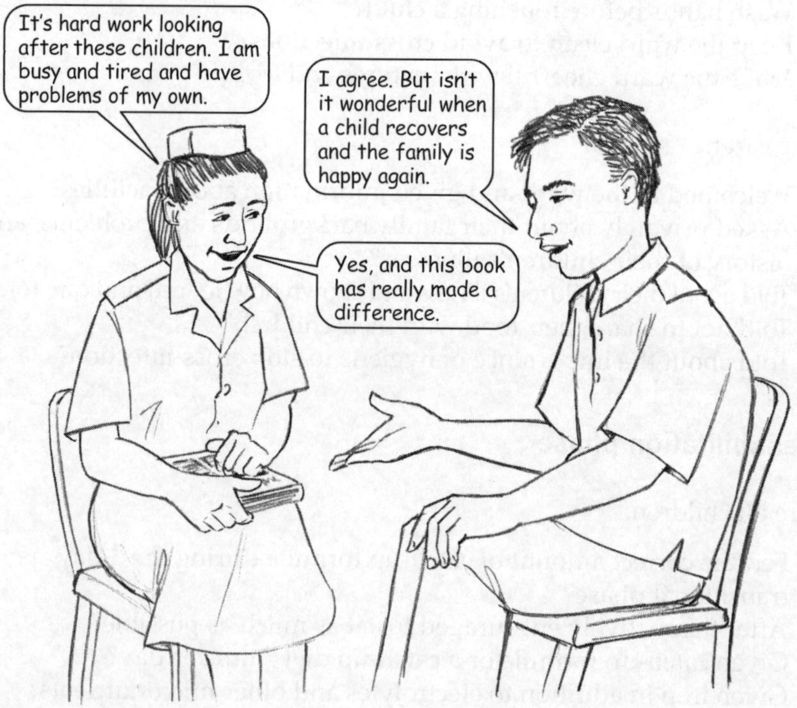

Figure 30 Caring for malnourished children is satisfying when done correctly.

Appendix

E Useful books and other resources

Contact the distributor or supplier for up-to-date prices. Single copies of books and print materials are sometimes sent free to developing country workers.

Note that this book is available as a CD-Rom from TALC.

Addresses

- **FANTA**: Food and Nutrition Technical Assistance Project, Academy for Educational Development, 1825 Connecticut Ave, Washington DC 20009, USA. fanta@aed.org
- **Nutriset**, BP 35-76770 Malaunay, France. nutriset@nutriset.fr
- Public Health Nutrition Unit, **London School of Hygiene and Tropical Medicine**, 49–51 Bedford Square, London WC1B 3DP, UK. ann.hill@lshtm.ac.uk
- **TALC**: Teaching-aids At Low Cost, PO Box 49, St Albans AL1 5TX, UK. talc@talcuk.org
- **Task Force SIGHT & LIFE**, Box 2116, 4002 Basel, Switzerland. sight.life@roche.com
- Public Health Programme, **University of the Western Cape**, Private Bag X17, Belville 7535, South Africa. tpuoane@uwc.ac.za
- **WHO**: World Health Organization, Ave Appia, 1211 Geneva 27, Switzerland. publications@who.ch

Books

Management of severe malnutrition: a manual for physicians and other senior health workers. WHO, 1999. Available from WHO.

Management of the child with a serious infection or severe malnutrition: guidelines for care at the first referral level in developing countries. WHO, 2000. Available from WHO or TALC.

A critical link: interventions for physical growth and psychological development. WHO, 1999. Available from WHO.

Guidebook on vitamin A in health and disease. 2nd edn. D. McLaren and M. Frigg, 2001. Available from Task Force Sight & Life, Switzerland.
Complementary feeding: family foods for breastfed children. WHO, 2000. Available from WHO.
HIV/AIDS: a guide to nutrition, care and support. FANTA, 2001. Available from FANTA.
Relactation: review of experience and recommendations for practice. WHO, 1998. Available from WHO.

Training courses

Improving the management of severe malnutrition: a training guide. A. Ashworth, T. Puoane, D. Sanders and C. Schofield, 2001. Available from London School of Hygiene and Tropical Medicine and University of the Western Cape.
Training course on the management of severe malnutrition. WHO, 2002. Available from WHO Regional Offices or, for Europe, from Dr Sultana Khanum, WHO, Geneva. khanums@who.ch

CD Roms and websites

Topics in international health: Nutrition. Wellcome Trust, 1999. Available from CABI Publishing, Wallingford, OX10 8DE, UK publishing@cabi.org or 10 E 40th St, Suite 3203, New York, NY 10016, USA cabi-nao@cabi.org
Teaching programme for severe malnutrition. www.capgan.org/unical.htm

Slides

Treatment of severely malnourished children. C. Schofield, A. Ashworth and A. Burgess, 2000. Available from TALC.
Undernutrition in young children. F. Savage and J. Copeman, 1998. Available from TALC.

Index

Note: page numbers in *italics* refer to illustrations